SECOND
THOUGHTS

PROVERBS 19: 2

SECOND THOUGHTS

Dr. Paul Simpson

THOMAS NELSON PUBLISHERS
Nashville • Atlanta • London • Vancouver

Published in Nashville, Tennessee, by Thomas Nelson, Inc., Publishers, and distributed in Canada by Word Communications, Ltd., Richmond, British Columbia, and in the United Kingdom by Word (UK), Ltd., Milton Keynes, England.

Unless otherwise noted, all Scripture quotations are from the New King James Version of the Bible, © 1979, 1980, 1982 by Thomas Nelson, Inc., Publishers.

Quotations marked NIV are from The Holy Bible: NEW INTERNATIONAL VERSION. Copyright © 1978 by the New York International Bible Society. Used by permission of Zondervan Publishers.

Scriptures quotations noted KJV are from The Holy Bible, King James Version.

Library of Congress Cataloging-in-Publication Data

Simpson, Paul, psychologist.
  Second thoughts / Paul Simpson
    p. cm.
  Includes bibliographical references.
  ISBN 0-7852-7418-9 (pbk.)
  1. False memory syndrome—Popular works. I. Title.
  RC455.2.F35S56   1997
  616.89—dc21   96-48196
                                    CIP

Printed in the United States of America

1 2 3 4 5 6 7 - 00 99 98 97

Dedication

This book is dedicated to victims of the "Witch Hunt," past and present. More than any person in history, God knows what it is to be falsely accused, to be humiliated and robbed of justice. From His own experience He stands beside each and every one of you—there is not a single victim of the Hunt that has escaped His sight. In the end His grace and justice will bring you vindication. In the end He will make all things right.

Contents

Preface

Joe, a newspaper reporter, is young and sharp, with an air of professionalism. Sitting across from me in my office, our conversation borders on the ludicrous. It would be comical, but we both know the topic of our conversation is deadly serious. He's heard about this "false memory" thing. Like so many others, he assumes that the stories of repression are true. But he's heard that I treat people recovering from false memories and wants to know more. He eyes me suspiciously, "Don't you think false memory syndrome is simply a result of fundamentalists denying the reality of abuse?" I have to smile: he really is new to this. I take his questions one by one, and watch his face grow more skeptical. He's not been exposed to the world of recovered memory therapy, and understandably, he finds the claims to be outlandish. "Could what you're describing be happening in modern America?" He takes me up on my offer to learn more about the False Memory Crisis. In the next year he meets dozens of accused families, regression believers, retractors, and professionals from across the nation. Murders, rapes, previous-lives traumas, the believers spill out their lurid tales of horror that they've recovered and their redemption found at the guiding hand of their therapists. He also hears the other side—the destroyed families and the survivors of these outlandish "therapies." At the end of the year he writes a stunning three-part exposé. Each day the issue is carried on the front page of the Arizona Daily Star and continued for two complete pages inside. With honest, straightforward reporting, the series uncovers the absurdities and abuses of the recovered memory movement. An entire city was suddenly forced to come to grips with what was happening in their very midst, under the guise of "therapy."

Our culture has become obsessed with victimization. Bookstores have entire sections devoted to the subject. Television and radio programs showcase a long parade of victims from every imaginable affliction. Thousands of therapists and support groups offer up a smorgasbord of hardships to recover from. Whereas at one time we minimized abuses in our nation, now it seems we just can't get enough. It appears that anyone who claims the title of victim is assumed to be truthful and is granted special status and license. They're able to hate, rage, and accuse because, after all, they're the victim.

In the middle of all this, the recovered memory movement has sprung up and become one of the strongest contributors to victim culture. For the last twenty years we've simply assumed that recovered memories reflected real events—it was a given. Its advocates got the "star treatment"—they made the talk show circuit, were featured in magazine and news articles, wrote bestsellers and became lecturers and "trauma experts." But somewhere in all the excitement we lost sight of some basic questions. "Could some of the recovered memories possibly be false?" "Does hypnosis really unlock repressed traumas?" "What about the accused's side of the story?" Proverbs 18:17 warns us, "The first to present his case seems right, till another comes forward and questions him" (NIV). In the beginning, Joe was well versed in one side of the story. It was only as he allowed himself to hear the other side that he found a balanced perspective. Since 1993 I've been sharing "the other side" with thousands in various professions, the media and the general public. Learning about "the other side" is what this book is all about.

I'll make my confession to you from the very start. I'm not a crusader by desire or design. My passion is in the art and science of psychology—reaching out to others, listening, counseling, learning, teaching, and healing. Personally, my own inclination is to stay out of conflicts, be safe, have a quiet little practice, provide for my family, and keep them out of harm's way. But something has happened that has broken my quiet pursuits. That "something" is arguably the most important family, psychological and theological issue of our time. Within these pages is my own story of deception, deliverance and redemption. But more importantly this book reflects the quiet horror of thousands who have been swept into one of the greatest hysterias of this century, a magnitude not seen since the last cycles of the great Witch Hunts.

At times I feel a bit like Moses standing before the burning bush, "'O Lord, please send someone else to do it,' There are those more eloquent and intelligent. Let them sound the alarm, take up the cause. I'm happy in my quiet little corner." There's a natural hesitation to write down an account of my own foolishness and then place it before the world to see, critique and mock. There are so many rationalizations that my mind and cowardice bring up, hoping the excuses will somehow stick. But the truth be told, there are few who are more experienced in working with regression believers, the devastated families and bewildered retractors. Through Project Middle Ground, I have found myself in the very heat of the battle—mediating between families and accusing adult children, offering restoration counseling to retractors, and doing educational seminars for professionals and the general public. And therein lies the dilemma. There is too much I've seen and learned. For me to be silent is to give quiet, passive approval to the "Hunt." That is not an option.

So I write to you out of moral imperative. Simply put, what is happening in the False Memory Crisis is wrong, horrifically wrong. While my own selfish inclinations take me in the opposite direction, my conscience gives me clear counsel. History teaches that we are not challenged to take a moral stand when it is convenient. To the contrary, it seems people are called upon at the most inopportune times—mid-career, to the threat of family and self, against the tide of popular thought and sentiment, at the cost of life, liberty and reputation.

But before I sound too much like a martyr, allow me to point out that thousands of believers in the recovered memory movement have already experienced far greater losses. Their life-shattering stories of misguided therapy and unspeakable psychological torture are captured in the pages to come. But the tragedy does not end with them. Thousands of accused families have also been devastated beyond comprehension—having lost children, grandchildren, careers, reputations, marriages, life savings, even having been falsely imprisoned. The true cost of the False Memory Crisis has been borne upon the shoulders of recovered memory believers and their families, written in their blood. I am simply bearing witness to their tragedy.

The product of more than three years of thought and articulation, this book seeks to give you a readable, accessible description of the issues involved in the False Memory Crisis and is drawn from a reasoned and experienced base of knowledge. I have purposely moved away from a "textbookish" writing style, but this has been tempered by the need to present complex issues clearly. Knowledge is power. The more informed you are, the less vulnerable you are to the claims, theories and misleading teachings found within the recovered memory movement. But be forewarned, with knowledge comes responsibility. Beyond simply learning about the False Memory Crisis, you may find that you are called to act upon that knowledge as well.

A word regarding things spiritual and scientific. I am bilingual, a faithful citizen of two countries. As a Christian and a Scientist I find that the two realms I belong to sometimes war against each other, cursing and throwing dispersions in a native tongue the other does not understand. Often they look on the other with contempt—certain that those who speak differently are stupid and uninformed. But fortunately, I am not alone in my dual citizenship. There are many like myself. We understand that ultimately there is a single kingdom, and a single King. He has given us both languages, Theology and Science, to explore and understand the world He has created. I've written *Second Thoughts* in such a way that those who do not identify with the Christian faith will be able to read this book with little offense. At the same time, I've made sure that the Christian perspective is addressed, particularly in Chapter Eleven. Despite my precautions, there will be those who object to my speaking the other language. Christians who will wonder why I bother with all that psychobabble nonsense and scientists who scoff that I would entertain the notions of a loving God and the real nature of evil. To both sides I offer no apologies. But I do offer an invitation: come and learn. Join me in the pursuit of truth that is found between the extremes.

I have spent my career working with those who have been abused as well as perpetrators of abuse. As a trauma specialist I am well-versed in the issues these populations present. But in coming to terms with the False Memory Crisis I've had to expand my vision to include those who have been falsely accused and victims of fraudulent therapies. There will be those who object from one extreme or the other. "Pro-victim" therapists who will wonder why I dare to question the abuse of anyone, anywhere. "Pro-accused" who will wonder why I wasn't more forceful in my statements, that I continue to account for true victims of abuse. Coming to terms with the False Memory Crisis is not an "either/or" proposition, it is both. Real abuse of children is occurring. But families are being falsely accused of horrific crimes based on recovered "memories." The only thing that compares to the horror of child abuse is to be falsely accused of these crimes. But in society's rush to judgment, the basic human right to be presumed innocent until proven guilty has often been lost. We are charged with an awesome task of finding balance, and we can accept nothing less.

Outline of *Second Thoughts*

Here's a brief overview of how the book is set up:

Chapters One, Two, and Three are designed to give you a basic understanding of the recovered memory movement.

Chapters Four, Five, and Six explore how remembering and forgetting occur, the evidence for the existence of multigenerational satanists, and the use of "symptoms" of repressed traumas.

Chapter Seven describes my own personal turning point, explores the basics of False Memory Syndrome and introduces you to "retractors."

Chapters Eight, Nine, and Ten explore possible contributors to false memories, including therapists' leading, misuse of hypnosis, suggestive readings, toxic group dynamics, Fantasy Prone Personalities, Grade Five Syndrome, personality disorders, certain types of mental illness and "effort after meaning."

Chapter Eleven evaluates the recovered memory movement in light of Scripture and traditional Christian teaching.

Finally, Chapter Twelve looks to the future and explores the decline of regressionism, the plight of its promoters, and the challenges we all face.

As you read through the chapters, here are a couple of points to keep in mind:

One of the things you'll notice is the regular use of feminine pronouns ("she," "hers") when I'm talking about clients active in the recovered memory movement. This is done for a basic reason. Research is consistent in showing those in the movement are somewhere between 92 percent to 97 percent women. Accordingly, it would be misleading for me to suggest that regression believers are equally men and women.

When discussing my clients' stories or using their quotes it is important to protect their identity. So I've used pseudonyms and altered specific details about their lives in order to protect them. When I've done this you'll notice their names are in quotes the first time I use them (e.g. "Mary" shares about her first week in therapy . . .). This lets you know this is a pseudonym. If a story has already been cited in the media then I am at liberty to use the person's real name.

Finally, the recovered memory movement generates extremely graphic sexual, violent images in it's believers. Accordingly you'll find that some sections contain disturbing accounts. This wasn't done to sensationalize the stories, I wanted to make sure that I accurately represented victims of the False Memory Crisis. Where possible I've toned down the stories or deleted obscene references. But be forewarned that some accounts may prove to be offensive nonetheless.

Acknowledgments

My deepest appreciation to Christy Voelkel for her many hours of writing, editing, and wise feedback. The project never would have been completed without her help and patience. Many thanks to my editors, Rick Nash, Melanee Bandy, and Cindy Blades, who were instrumental in guiding and shaping this project. My appreciation to Eric Nelson and Scott Richards for their help during the early drafts. To Linda Ross, your gracious spirit and courage have been a welcome influence in my life.

My thanks to the reviewers who took the time to critique earlier drafts. This includes Diana Anderson, Chuck Brainerd, Tom Copps, Ronald Enroth, Pamela Freyd, Elizabeth Loftus, Paul McHugh, Gene Moan, Jeff Parziale, Gretchen and Bob Passantino, and Cindy Ward.

Over the years I have had the privilege to be mentored by some extraordinary human beings. I am indebted for the many gifts they have given—without their contributions I would have lacked the critical thinking and tools that have proved so essential. To Darrald Vaughn for his firm guiding hand and godly character. Betty Newlon for teaching the "duck-walk," a contagious laughter and courage for life. Kevin Leman for teaching a new dog old tricks and his ongoing encouragement and guidance. To John Bloom for his loving, humorous, and compassionate nature. To Gene Moan, a role model and living, breathing example of Christian and professional integrity. To Ralph Earle, your professionalism and vulnerable honesty set the standard for me. My deepest thanks to each of you.

To Diana Anderson, Laura Pasley and Cindy Ward. Each of you have been selfless trail-blazers in the retractor community and have played such an important role in teaching me the flesh-and-blood side of the False Memory Crisis. I deeply appreciate and value your friendship.

To Erin, my partner and very best friend, for your continuous sacrifice, humor, support and encouragement that has allowed this book to become a reality. Thank you for the dance of a lifetime, I am privileged to spend it with you. To Maizie and Woody for being who you are. You bring joy, laughter and deep satisfaction into your Papa's life. I am so very proud of each of you.

To Mary Simpson, for your belief and dedication throughout the years. Your godly walk and strength of character have been a constant role model for me to follow, Su Aga Po. To Woodley Simpson, one of the greatest men I have ever known. Your nature and strength lives on within me. You are missed.

Set on the soul's acropolis the reason stands
A virgin, arm'd, commercing with celestial light,
And he who sins against her has defiled his own Virginity:
No cleansing makes his garment white;
So clear is reason. But how dark, imagining,
Warm, dark, obscure and infinite, daughter of Night:
Dark is her brow, the beauty of her eyes with sleep
Is loaded, and her pains are long, and her delight.

C. S. LEWIS, "REASON," *POEMS*, 1964[1]

1

Second Thoughts

We are so constituted that we believe the most incredible things; and, once they are engraved upon the memory, woe to him who would endeavor to erase them.

GOETHE, *THE SORROWS OF YOUNG WERTHER*, 1774

"Mary's" voice on the phone was quiet and distant. The first thing she let me know was that she didn't trust me, or any other therapist for that matter. The only reason she had called was because she had heard that I worked with people who were trying to come out of regression therapy.

"I'm not sure what's true anymore. The memories feel so real, but I'm beginning to have doubts. I really care about my therapist, and she's warned me about people like you, those who question the reality of recovered memories. But I'm at a breaking point. I'm thinking of taking my life because I can't take the pain. I just don't know what's real anymore."

I responded as honestly as I knew how. "Mary, whatever you do, don't trust me. Allow yourself to have questions, to be skeptical, to use your mind once more. Let's talk, but you need to stay in the driver's seat."

A series of long-distance phone calls followed.

Mary shared, "What happened? That's part of the pain, not knowing when things got messed up and out of control, when an innocent cry for help turned into permission for someone to rape your soul, mind, and heart. It's so frustrating, so humiliating, and so bizarre."

The cycle had started two years earlier, when Mary began having problems in her marriage.

"The whole thing started with requests for prayer. I turned, as I have done so many times, to prayer, to God. I asked others to pray, some friends even fasted. In a Bible study the teacher asked us to pray and ask the Lord to help us identify anything that might be a barrier in our lives to intimacy with God. Afterward, in a conversation with that teacher, I shared about the troubles in my marriage. She prayed and said that the Lord was impressing upon her that I was sexually abused as a child. As I began to weep, she held me like Mom would have, if she hadn't been two thousand

3

miles away. She then revealed that she was a counselor and wanted me at her house the next day to start working through this revelation."

Trusting her Christian leader, hurting, looking for answers— Mary never guessed that she was about to embark on a dark descent into the world of "regressionism."

"The next day was the first of many sessions involving inner child therapy, visualization, and 'chair work.' We even visualized (with the Lord's help) my father being abused by the grandfather who was in my memories, and then my father abusing my mother. There's no way I could have known about these events, but there really weren't any boundaries to this madness. I did lots of writing, lots of introspection into wrongs done by others to me—some actual, some 'recovered.' There were rape, incest, hatred, sodomy, we even remembered the words they spoke as they did these evil things. The work was hard. But it was also stimulating, challenging. I had embarked on a journey few had traveled—the counselor said I had the worst case of sexual abuse she had ever seen and that I was one of her hardest workers. I was proud. She also told me I didn't have to tell anyone what we had learned in our sessions, including my husband or parents. In fact, she said I really shouldn't say anything to anyone until I didn't care whether people believed me or not. A secret! Somehow I felt special."

Mary's thinking became more distorted.

"I was being acknowledged as the poor victim. There was attention, there was sympathy, there was empathy. I could finally stand on the table like a spoiled three-year-old and scream, 'Look what they did' and even be praised for the hard work I was doing. I was transcending to a place where I was God—if I used the tools I was shown, if I accepted the truth I had remembered, if I didn't falter. Then I could not only find this Nirvana, but reign as supreme there. I delved 100 percent into the quest for Nirvana in all the other areas of my life, areas that weren't even really a problem until I went through this counseling. I was determined that if I did it right, I could be in control of my life and do as good a job as God did, if not better. And that's what I did. Not surprisingly, disappointment and shame came quickly. I couldn't be God—how angry and ashamed I was. It was so frustrating. My counselor was doing it—why couldn't I?"

She gradually grew more distant from family and friends.

"By now I was being careful not to get too close to my family; in fact I had pushed them away. I was suspicious of my husband because I was told he must be as 'sick' as I was since he married me. All the while I was riddled with shame for the many failures I was committing daily. I had resolved myself to the fact that I was going to be a failure forever, in everything. I was one of the fortunate ones who now had the therapeutic tools, but I just wasn't 'good enough' to make them work. What was wrong with me?"

As Mary's despair deepened, she took the forbidden step of sharing what was happening with old friends who weren't part of her "therapy."

"My friends outside of regression therapy were increasingly stunned the more I talked. They didn't seem to understand the great act of betrayal I was committing just by talking to them. Because of their questioning and unbelief, I began to wonder. Meanwhile, a friend in my regression therapy had just issued a permanent restraining order against her parents because of things she had recovered."

"With the help of outside friends, I finally told my mom what had gone on in the last eighteen months of my life. She and Dad were so supportive, so loving, and so willing to help however they could. I was hurting so badly. Something inside was dying. Mom said it sounded worse than amnesia because I remembered things that might or might not be true. She told me that my therapy sounded like date rape—I had trusted and was then betrayed by someone saying she loved me."

That's when Mary made the decision to call me. Like tens of thousands of people, Mary had been led into regressionism step by step, never guessing that this therapy would lead to sick dependency and wild delusions. Her therapist was a Christian and trusted by Mary's church. The attention, acceptance, and praise Mary received from her felt wonderful. But the price tag was more then she bargained for. The promised healing never materialized. Mary had been convinced that it couldn't be the therapist's fault—she was too knowledgeable and perfect. It had to be Mary's fault—she needed to try harder, come up with just one more image, one more breakthrough. But Nirvana was never forthcoming.

In Mary's groups, no one was ever allowed to doubt the memories created through regression "science" and the leading of the "Holy Spirit." The theories were presented as unwavering facts, and any who questioned the process were "in denial" about the reality of abuse. But for the first time in a year and a half, Mary was able to ask the questions that had been forbidden by her leader and group members. She was at last able to hear another perspective and become educated about the myths she had been taught. Whenever possible, I provided her with original sources of research so that she could check things out for herself. Mary had been well indoctrinated, but she was finally able to break out of her mental straitjacket and begin the exhilarating journey back to reason and truth, back to thinking for herself. Mary is one of the lucky ones. Because of caring friends and family, she was able to find her way back out to reality, but so many have yet to do so. Instead they continue their descent into regressionism at an unspeakable cost.

Regression Therapy: The Fountain of Youth

We've all read the articles, watched the news briefs, and skimmed the inflammatory headlines in the grocery lines. A popular comedienne accuses her parents of having sexually abused her, publicly declaring vivid memories of her mother abusing her from infancy until she was six or seven years old, memories that she recovered after they lay dormant for years. Later she discovered that she had developed "multiple personalities" in order to cope with her trauma. A national magazine carries the story on its front cover.[2]

A former Miss America travels the country sharing her father's incredible sexual and physical abuses, events which she alleges she never recalled until she was an adult. In order to survive she split into a "day child," who giggled and smiled, and a "night child," who was regularly raped by her father. Her day child had no knowledge of the night child until she was twenty-four years old. Then the horrific images spilled forth.[3] Again, the story is carried on the front cover of a national magazine, for millions to read. These popular and riveting stories of forgotten abuse have seeped into the American consciousness and helped create the uneasy fear that any appearance of a normal, happy family life is only an empty facade fraught with hidden pain and memories.

Is Truth Stranger Than Fiction?

Stories of recovered memories share a common link. Along with graphic details that would strain the imagination of the most unscrupulous producer of B-grade slasher films, the victims claim to have experienced a form of selective amnesia. Unable to cope

with the shame and horror of their experiences, each has suc-
ceeded in repressing all memory of these events into a dark and
almost inaccessible corner of his or her unconscious mind. There
these memories have stayed, locked away from personal awareness until the victim sought the help of an increasingly popular
form of treatment called *regression therapy*. Thrust into the public
spotlight by best-selling books and a growing parade of syndi-
cated TV talk shows, popular magazines, and newspaper
accounts, regression therapy has made quite a splash in the mar-
ketplace of ideas. Advocates have portrayed this technique as a
powerful healing tool, with an ability to provide unprecedented
help for a vast array of personal problems.

One inpatient psychiatric program ran an ad in a national magazine that captures the promise of regression therapy:
"Remembering incest and childhood abuse is the first step to healing. We can help you remember and heal."[4] How can people know
if regression therapy is right for them? You could be a candidate,
the ad suggested, if you suffer from

> Mood swings, panic disorder, substance abuse, rage, flashbacks,
> depression, hopelessness, anxiety, paranoia, low self-esteem,
> relapse, relationship problems, sexual fear, sexual compulsion,
> self-mutilation, borderline personality, irritable bowel,
> migraine, P.M.S., post-traumatic stress, bulimia, anorexia,
> A.C.O.A. (Adult Children of Alcoholics), obesity, multiple per-
> sonality, hallucinations, religious addiction, parenting prob-
> lems, suicidal feelings.[5]

So what's the most effective course of treatment for these symptoms? "What we do best is help bring up forgotten memories
through our powerful combination of massage, body work, hypnosis, psychodrama, and sodium brevitol interviewing."[6]

The message of this marketing strategy is abundantly clear.
Nearly every personal problem, from a psychotic breakdown to
irregularity, can supposedly be healed by regression therapy.
Under the watchful care of a trained hospital staff and for tens of
thousands of dollars, every patient can expect miraculous results.
Deeply buried memories of sexual abuse and incest are identified
by these "trauma experts" as the culprit, with surprisingly little
room for variation. From thousands of miles away, they are able to
determine that a patient has repressed memories of abuse. One
size fits all, no waiting.

Where There's Smoke . . .

But *regressionists* (therapists who subscribe to regression doctrine) don't always agree as to what direction the symptoms point. One group is certain that a person's problems are a result of repressed childhood sexual trauma. But another group is equally certain that similar signs indicate ritual abuses by multigenerational satanists. They've developed elaborate conspiracy theories in which there are thousands of secret satanists in powerful positions who are killing countless children and adults in barbaric, ancient rituals. A growing number of women who are being identified with multiple personalities are the alleged survivors of these ritual tortures. Other regressionists can point a client in another direction to equally fertile soil for the roots of personal dysfunction. Brian Weiss, an East Coast psychiatrist, claims to have helped thousands of patients reexperience their past lives through his use of regression techniques. "People are having experiences: dreams, deja vus, spontaneous regressions. . . . I have a lot of psychiatrists, but also psychologists and other therapists, who call or write to me and tell me that they've been doing this work secretly or privately for the past 10 or 15 years, don't tell anyone, and out come these beautiful case histories."[7]

The psychiatrist is correct in his observation. In fact, nationally 28 percent of therapists believe that "hypnosis can be used to recover accurate memories of past lives."[8] An organization devoted to past-life therapy, The Association of Past-Life Research and Therapy, was formed in 1980 for "the protection of the people doing the work, and to have other people to talk to and share experiences with."[9] Glowing testimonials advance the theory that the discovery of past life-traumas enables us to better understand present-day pain. A prime-time investigative television program reported on this "therapy" and noted that this psychiatrist has a waiting list of nearly two thousand hopeful clients.[10]

Yet another group of regression believers maintains that the same "symptoms" indicate a person has been victimized by space aliens, but has repressed the trauma. John Mack, a Harvard professor, psychiatrist, and Pulitzer Prize-winning biographer, is concerned about the plight of space-alien abductees. "It does seem bizarre, but this is not the product of mental illness. These people speak genuinely about something powerful that has happened to them, and the feelings they bring—the terrors, sweats and body shakes—are real."[11] Many of his clients don't want to believe that they've been alien-abducted. But after therapy sessions that include hypnotic regression, clients are able to discover the "truth" of their victimization. "I am as careful as I know how to be in my diagnostic discriminations. I have exhausted all the possibilities that are purely psychological, even psychosocial, that could account for this."[12] One of Mack's clients, Joe, suddenly remembered his alien abduction two years before while he was getting physical therapy for a sore neck. Joe said, "I was no longer on the massage table, but on a cold table surrounded by extraterrestrials who were putting a needle in my neck. I had this incredible fear and this excruciating pain. Then, wham! I was back on the massage table."[13]

More abduction memories followed, including floating out of the window in his bedroom at two years of age and a prior life in which Joe was an alien. Joe declared: "I've gone through the terror and found incredible liberation on the other side. We need to treat this with an open mind. We can't keep saying we're the only intelligent species in the universe. We have to wake up."[14]

Another client of Mack's is a thirty-two-year-old clerical worker and mother of three. "Jerry" has been abducted over fifty times since she was a child. "I'm awakened by a tap. I feel paralyzed but awake. They invade you entirely. Then they float you out and up into the ship."[15] At first, she says, the aliens were her friends, but later they began doing painful gynecological experiments, including inserting embryos and extracting fetuses. This led to the birth of at least two alien children, whom she later met. She sought Dr. Mack for help. "I was hoping he would say I was crazy. Then I would know it wasn't real and I could be helped."[16] But Mack assured her she was not alone. Jerry, along with her three children, is now part of Mack's monthly support group for space alien abductees. She stated: "I'm not crazy; this is real. Who would want to make up a story like this?"[17]

Mack is certainly right on one point. His clients are not alone in their beliefs. Thousands of people are recounting memories of abduction by space aliens and (with chilling similarity to one another) are describing terrifying experiences of being rendered powerless and undergoing degrading, painful scientific examinations by otherworldly creatures. A recent Roper survey proclaimed that two out of every one hundred people have been space alien-abducted (that's over one hundred million people worldwide).[18] The problem is that most people don't remember their space alien trauma, though they have the symptoms. But with the help of caring professionals like Mack, people are able to recover their repressed memories.

But wait, there's more! Another emerging group of regression-ists claims that life's difficulties can be traced back to traumatic events a person experienced in the womb. Recently, I was interviewed on *Frontline*, an investigative program on PBS, for which I was commenting on the questionable practices of regression therapists. In one segment a group therapy session was shown in which a therapist was regressing a group member back in time, to the point that she found the client had been stuck in the fallopian tube of her mother. With great tears and drama, the therapist helped the client through the fallopian tube, where she could then find her way to the father's sperm and become implanted in the womb. The therapist explained, "People, as I said, they're here to heal and, in the process, they can go as far back as their own psyche will allow them, their own consciousness will allow them to go. . . . There are some people that go even beyond conception, like the woman that accessed a memory from when she was in the fallopian tube and got stuck and this stuckness has hurt her in her adult life. . . . And so when she is able to change that in some way, she can move forward with ease in her life. And that needs to be corrected at the source of the problem, which for her was in the fallopian tube."[19]

Nationally, 54 percent of therapists believe that memories can be retrieved from infancy.[20] In fact, an inpatient program in California offers, for the right price, to take you back to the fetal state to reexperience hurtful things that your parents said about you. A recent episode of *The Oprah Winfrey Show* featured "regressed-womb" clients who gave glowing testimonials about how dramatically their lives have improved since they were able to return to the womb and hear the horrible things their parents had said while they were still *in utero*.[21]

The personal testimonies of those whose lives have been touched by regression therapy are legion. Some of their stories speak of ritual abuse, others of reincarnation or abduction by extraterrestrials. Tragically, many of these traumatic memories have resulted in public character assassination and the destruction of thousands of families. Successful lawsuits based on "recovered memories" have awarded millions for harm done by alleged ritual and sexual abusers and even imprisonment for some of the accused (see examples in Chapter 12.)

With such a flood of witnesses coming forward to make these claims, it would be easy to conclude that something *is* happening in our midst. After all, where there's smoke, there's fire. But the troubling fact is, corroborating evidence of these traumatic memories is consistently lacking. When evaluated in the cold light of objective reality, claims of recovered memories of years of sexual torture, an epidemic of satanic abuse, UFO abductions, or past-life traumas are weak and subjective at best. In fact, the mounting evidence is to the contrary. With a chilling awakening, many are coming to understand that sometimes where there's smoke, there's just smoke.

Needless to say, the claims, counterclaims, and the sensationalistic nature of regression therapy have created the hottest debate in psychology in decades. It's called the False Memory Crisis. Adding to the furor is the fact that a cottage industry has grown up around this practice, featuring inpatient treatment programs, books, and talk-show circuits. Thousands of therapists have been trained in, and use, regression techniques. One study showed that 71 percent of doctoral-level psychologists have made use of regression techniques in an effort to recover repressed memories in clients.[22] Countless seminars each year teach the theory of repression as fact and offer the latest methods of regressing clients. Journals have been established to explore patients' horrific stories of repressed abuse by parents, satanists, space aliens, and perpetrators from centuries ago. Make no mistake about it, regressionism is a big-ticket item.

The high-stakes nature of this controversy is evident. But are genuinely hurting people finding a newly discovered key to personal healing? Or is a desperate and gullible public being led to a therapeutic dead end, paved with personal destruction, trashed reputations, and destroyed family relationships?

A Front-Row Seat

At the outset I have to admit that no one would be less likely to raise questions than I. As a former case manager for Child Protective Services and now as a psychologist in private practice, I've worked extensively with victims of physical and sexual abuse and the perpetrators who abused them. These experiences have provided me a front-row seat to display after display of the extreme cruelty people are capable of committing. But I've also seen the beautiful resiliency of the human spirit in enduring and overcoming barbaric levels of evil.

Through the day-to-day experiences of my counseling practice I had become accustomed to listening to stories of abuse, but several years ago I began to notice the emergence of a significant trend. I encountered a growing number of clients who reported memories of abuse that had been "repressed" for decades until they had been brought back to light through different hypnotic techniques.

Given my areas of specialty, I wanted to find out more about this dramatic new tool in the fight against abuse. I eagerly attended several seminars where I was taught regression techniques and theory. Under the supervision of a nationally known regressionist, I furthered my training. Since I already had a background in hypnosis, I was quickly able to incorporate regression therapy into my counseling practice. With the very best of intentions, I began to use these techniques with my clients, and sure enough, they began to recover images of sexual abuse and other terrifying crimes that had been committed against them.

At the time I was also working at an inpatient psychiatric hospital, where patients were being regressed to uncover their forgotten abuses. From a personal and professional point of view, the experience was anything but encouraging. I watched grown women and men turn into crying, incoherent, psychotic personalities. Clutching teddy bears, balled up in the corner of their rooms, these patients would talk with voices of five-year-olds. Their stories contained imaginative horrors ranging from being raped for years to bizarre accounts of being forced to murder and eat their own newborn children by powerful satanic cults.

But the more they pursued this new form of "healing," the more I watched their lives unravel. I was told repeatedly by "regression experts" that the psychotic episodes I observed in their patients were due to the intensity of recovered traumas. The notion that regression techniques were actually the cause of the patient's deteriorated state was not even entertained as a possibility. At no time were we allowed to question their validity. With dictatorial zeal, they told us that the patients' hypnotic images could only be interpreted as reality, no matter how outlandish or impossible they might seem. Critical evaluation was seen as further persecution of a helpless victim.

The raging and babbling were only the beginning. The patients discharged from the hospital were usually prescribed volumes of psychiatric medications. Later, many had to be readmitted to the hospital because of suicide attempts, cutting themselves with razors, or simply being unable to survive out in the real world. Many of these patients had a lifetime of high achievements: straight As in school, advanced college degrees, and stellar success in business. These formerly high-functioning individuals were now unable to keep their jobs, leave their homes, or care for their children. Divorces followed as once strong families splintered apart.

Again and again it was stressed that the disintegration of these patients' lives was due to the traumas they had incurred decades ago. After years of stable routine, raising families, and building successful careers, the "truth" had finally come to light. Their violent repudiation of a comforting facade of normalcy was the first step to recovery. I watched and waited, but oddly, the promised recovery was never forthcoming. The patients attended increasing amounts of individual and group therapy, immersed themselves in reading about recovery and repression, went through multiple hospitalizations, and yet where was the payoff? There was still no healing from the ailments that caused the patients to seek help in the first place. In fact, they were worse off mentally, physically, and socially than when they entered therapy.

The Disaster Spreads

Compounding this tragic state of affairs was that the pain of the regression experience would not be limited to the patient. As in any other black-and-white worldview, the heroes and villains were easy to spot. The patients were the heroes who finally found the courage to stand against monstrous evil. The villains in this story were mothers and fathers who were implicated in the patients' hypnotic images. Typically, they lived several states away and never had contact with the counseling staff. I discovered it's much easier to build a case if the accused never gets a hearing.

The family confrontation was inevitable. Complete detachment from one's perpetrators was an essential step to an "individuated," healthy life. Patients were trained extensively for the moment they would confront their parents with the discovered abuses and were told their perpetrators would be in denial when confronted. Therapists assisted patients in writing out long, angry letters that would eventually be read to the parents. Patients would practice reading the letters aloud to their therapists and support-group members. During these "encouragement" sessions, no one ever questioned whether the hypnotic images contained in the letters might be false, or suggested that the accused had a right to offer their own defense. The cardinal truth of regression therapy was driven home with unmistakable clarity: "The patient's emotional reality is all that matters." There was no option that allowed the parents to be innocent. In fact, denial by a patient's mother and father would be verification that they had actually committed the fantasized crimes.

When the unwitting parents were brought to the hospital, they could never have imagined the nightmare that awaited them. Brought into a room with their daughter and her therapist, they were told that they were to remain absolutely silent as she read her confrontation letter. At the end, the parents were allowed two options. They could confess that they were guilty of these horrific crimes and begin the long, arduous journey of recovery (typically facilitated by the same regressionist). The second option was to maintain their innocence, which would only mean they were "in denial" and guilty as charged but trying to cover up their crimes. The parents' shock and vehement rejection of the accusations were always interpreted as further evidence of their guilt.

As my practice of regressionism continued, my discomfort became more pronounced. It occurred to me that regression therapy hadn't been taught in any of my doctoral training. In the face of increasingly outlandish results, I discovered my only support for my beliefs and techniques were the sure dictates of "regression experts" and the pronouncements of pop-psychology books. At that point I made a personal commitment to better understand the regression phenomenon and went to the Arizona State University library and began what I thought would be a brief overview of the research. I knew that with a bit of scholarly reading I could lay my concerns to rest. But what I discovered had a profound impact on the "facts" I had been taught in the regression seminars and began for me a personal journey which continues to this day.

The Baby with the Bathwater

One of my greatest concerns as I started to doubt was, "What about someone who has really been abused—am I denying the reality of his or her trauma?" There was a danger that I was accidentally throwing out the baby with the bathwater, that is, denying actual cases of abuse in an effort to prevent false accusations from being made. But my nagging questions and doubts were pulling at me. I couldn't destroy the lives of innocent people in the name of identifying abusers. Truth matters. If a person has really been abused, the truth of his or her abuse is important. However, if someone has merely fantasized about being abused, that distinction needs to be made. Lives are hanging in the balance.

Table 1 is a practical way of grasping the important differences I'm talking about. This is a description of different categories of memory, suggested by Dr. Paul McHugh, director of psychiatry at Johns Hopkins University Medical School. Take a moment to look at each of the squares.

TABLE 1 Memory of Abuse
Reality of Abuse

	Abuse Happened	Abuse Didn't Happen
Remember	Remembered Abuse [abused and remembers]	False Alarm [no abuse but has memory]
Forget	Forgotten [abused but no memory]	Non-abused [no abuse and no memory]

The *Remembered Abuse* box describes people who have been truly abused and have always remembered their abuse. "Susan," a mother of three children, is sitting in my office. At the age of eight, she lived with her uncle and his family for a summer. What was supposed to have been a time of fun with cousins turned into a two-month nightmare. Her uncle's good-natured touches turned into uncomfortable caresses. Eventually, despite her protests, he became increasingly sexual with her. Susan was trapped and had no way of sharing her fear and disgust. She endured the humiliation of that summer and because of her deep shame vowed to never tell anyone her dark secret. The years passed, but the shame and harm never faded. In her quiet moments, Susan would sometimes allow her thoughts to turn to her abuse and desperately wished that there was a way to let out the pain bottled up inside her. Finally, at the age of thirty-eight, Susan decided that she couldn't bear her secret any longer. She entered therapy and the relief she found was tremendous. In counseling she broke her long silence and was able to resolve her issues of rage, shame, self-blaming, and grief.

At any point during those intervening years, Susan could freely recall the hurtful abuses by her uncle, but she chose not to deal with her trauma. These are *freestanding memories*, which are generally reliable. Freestanding memories of abuse are not involved in the False Memory Crisis. The reality of physical, emotional, and sexual abuse is all too frequent in cultures throughout the world, and no one should doubt that sexual abuse of children exists and produces suffering and long-term consequences. Victims like Susan have a right to pursue healing through competent therapy and deserve compassion and support. In fact, helping victims heal from their traumas has been the focus of much of my therapeutic career.

The next box down is *Forgotten*, and it refers to people who have been actual victims of abuse but have forgotten these events. As we'll discover in Chapter 4, all people forget large portions of their childhood, which can include hurtful events. This is also the square that regression patients see themselves in. As we'll see in Chapter 4, *forgetting* and *repressing* are very different concepts. Can someone forget something and remember it years later? Certainly. Can someone instantly and selectively repress a traumatic experience and moments later have no recollection of the event? Welcome to the controversy.

In the third square, *False Alarms* represent those who erroneously claim to have memories of abuse which have never happened. In scientific terms these people are referred to as *false positives*. It stands to reason that, of the thousands of claims of recovered memories of incest, ritual abuse, space-alien torture, and past-life traumas, some considerable portion is false. It is this portion that we refer to as *false memories*.

Finally, you'll see that the box in the lower right-hand corner is *Non-abused*. These are people who have never experienced physical or sexual abuse and correctly have no memories of such abuse. In practical terms, this square does not exist for regressionists. As

Roseanne Arnold noted on a talk show, "When someone asks you, 'Were you sexually abused as a child?' there are only two answers: One of them is 'Yes,' and one of them is 'I don't know.' You can't say 'No.'"[23] For regression believers, it is only the insightful workings of the regressionist that allows a person to really know whether or not he or she has been abused. *Remembered (freestanding), forgotten, false alarms,* and *non-abused* may sound like technical, abstract concepts, but they have real implications. *Notice that recognizing the reality of one square in no way diminishes the reality of another.* Even if some repressed memories are real, this does not invalidate the fact that false alarms are also occurring. And vice versa—false alarms don't invalidate true claims of abuse. In understanding the False Memory Crisis, I was challenged to find an important balance of recognizing the reality of abuse and acknowledging that false memories are occurring and hurting people. It wasn't an "either-or" proposition, it was "both."

None of the regressionists I knew (myself included) did anything to account for false alarms. We weren't alone. An astounding 57 percent of therapists nationally report they do nothing at all to differentiate truth from fiction when working with hypnotic images of abuse.[24] If people want to pay a hundred dollars an hour to fantasize about "past lives," they are free to do so, and the negative consequences upon other people in their lives are typically minimal. But when the consequences of a false alarm become more pronounced, our standard for accepting the accuracy of someone's abuse claims needs to be raised. In real terms this meant that some portion of the families I had helped accuse were innocent, but I hadn't incorporated any safety measures that would protect them.

The American Medical Association has grave concerns about recovered memories of abuse:

> Few cases in which adults make accusations of childhood sexual abuse based on recovered memories can be proved or disproved and it is not yet known how to distinguish true memories from imagined events in these cases. . . . The AMA considers recovered memories . . . of childhood sexual abuse to be of uncertain authenticity, which should be subject to external verification. The use of recovered memories is fraught with problems of potential misapplication.[25]

The Journey Begins

Proverbs 17:15 tells us, "Acquitting the guilty and condemning the innocent—the LORD detests them both" (NIV). We know that child abuse is a tragedy impacting many lives. Yet to be falsely accused of these crimes is equally as horrible. People are left without a defense for something that supposedly took place decades ago. Is it possible that both real abuse and false accusations are taking place within our society? The intent of this book is not to further traumatize actual victims. I want to share with you my journey of seeking for the truth and to provide you a basis for discernment and balance within the most pressing family issue of our time. How can this be done? A foundation of facts, reason, and science will assist us in examining this intensely controversial issue.

For the past twenty years, regressionism has been an increasingly popular movement that has left thousands of families and clients destroyed in its wake. Like other regressionists, I had intertwined my fervent beliefs in regression therapy around the issues related to actual victims of abuse. With the best of intentions, I had believed and taught the promises of regressionism, but I had failed to fully consider all the evidence or critically evaluate what I had been taught. Proverbs 19:2 warns us, "It is not good to have zeal without knowledge, nor to be hasty and miss the way" (NIV). Regressionists, myself included, have done both. The time has come for a closer examination.

This book is a description of my journey from doing regression therapy to eventually intervening in the False Memory Crisis. For me, the first steps in coming out of this movement began with my questioning the confident dictates and theories I had been taught. My search for the truth has led me to discussions with a wide spectrum of experts who treat multiple personality disorder, renowned psychiatrists, leading memory researchers, ground breaking attorneys, forensic psychologists, investigative reporters, cult investigators, retractors, clergymen, law-enforcement specialists in satanic ritual abuse cases, and the FBI. In the pages that follow, I want to share what I've learned along the way.

The journey begins.

The World of Regressionism

We (Americans) suffer primarily not from our vices or our weaknesses, but from our illusions. We are haunted, not by reality, but by those images we have put in place of reality.

DANIEL J. BOORSTIN, THE IMAGE, 1962

Our story opens as a crystal-clear voice swells over the darkened auditorium. Poised serenely on the lit stage, Ann pours golden notes over the expectant crowd. It's a senior music recital, and this moment celebrates a life of achievement, surrounded by a loving family, filled with festivity and comfort. And yet, in the midst of this, Ann, seemingly healthy and productive, feels alone and isolated from her mother. Two days after the recital, after a particularly painful telephone conversation, Ann sought counseling to help her grapple with the conflicts she had regarding their relationship. She found a regressionist who suggested that Ann may have been sexually abused as a child but had repressed the events. This opened the door to six years of regression therapy.

Early in her therapy, Ann claimed she had recently gone to a party where she was raped by an older man, which she said set off the strings of memories where she could "see" her father's face superimposed over that of the rapist. With the regressionist's help, Ann was able to go back in time to reexperience volumes of hidden sexual and physical trauma, and to acknowledge the denial she had been in for years. This culminated with Ann trying to kill herself and being admitted to a hospital. Then the regressionist confronted Ann's bewildered parents on the phone, firmly stating that they had abused their daughter. Neither the siblings nor the parents could remember any behavior even hinting of abuse, but for Ann and her regressionist this only verified the accusation. The family was "in denial" and would never get better until they acknowledged the truth.

Ann dropped out of life, quit her singing, lost most of her friends, and all of her family. With the help of the nurturing and persistent regression therapist and his hypnotic techniques, Ann dedicated herself to discovering her forgotten memories. Her search through the faint hallways of dusty images brought forth an ever-changing cast of family members in shifting roles and scenes. Gruesome details from satanic rituals involving Ann's entire family emerged, and she came to believe that she had at least twenty-seven different personalities living inside of her, each one clamoring for her attention, creating intense inner turmoil and dramatic suicide attempts. Her various "personalities" regularly cut and burned her, and she careened in and out of hospitals, riding a roller coaster of attempted suicides.

Eventually, following the advice of her regressionist, Ann unsuccessfully sued her parents and grandparents for twenty million dollars based on her fantasies of years of ritual abuse. They presented the specific cruelties gathered from her recovered images, which included the belief that these were not her biological parents but actually members of a satanic cult. Her pseudo-mother had sexually abused her with broomsticks, spiders, wires, and vegetables and by attaching electrodes to her genitals. Her pseudo-father had an assortment of hardware with which he sexually tortured her. He had also dropped her into a pool to drown, and forced her to watch ritual-related abortions.

The absurdity of the situation confounded the family. In order to combat the accusations, they brought in school records of perfect attendance and pediatrician records of a very healthy and unmarred little girl. They dug about in their own memories, trying to imagine how their relational difficulties might have affected a sensitive child. But none of this mattered in their attempt to shake their daughter's convictions. It didn't make any difference. The regressionist made no attempt to change Ann's perception of her newfound reality, as he felt that it would violate her trust and reinjure her.

What are the fruits of Ann's journey into regressionism? She has lost her musical career, is living on disability, and is alone except for her new family of regression believers. With unflinching faith in her horrific new memories, Ann lives with the firm conviction that she is a "survivor." Her parents' marriage cracked under the emotional and legal strain, ending in divorce. They and her siblings were divided and crushed under this blow. They have not had a relationship with Ann in years and have no hope of ever regaining one.

The regressionist continues with a thriving practice, each new client a potential "Ann" in the making. He firmly stands by Ann and her story. You see, he's a "trauma expert" who provides this treatment for many, many patients. He declares that when he is deposed in court he has no need to present corroborative evidence for a client's claims. What is most important, he believes, is the client's inner truth, regardless of what actually happened historically. He says that we all live in a delusion, that nobody really knows the truth. His beliefs echo the hollow philosophy of another man, a man who also abdicated his duty to protect the innocent. "What is truth?" he asked, and he washed his hands.[1]

Just What Is Repression?

"Repression." . . . The word whispers of dark secrets and buried treasures, of rooms filled with cobwebs and dust, with a strange unearthly rustling in the corners. Repression is the most haunting and romantic of concepts in the psychology of memory: Something happens, something so shocking and frightful that the mind short-circuits and the normal workings of memory go seriously awry. An entire memory, or perhaps a jagged piece of a memory, is split off and hidden away. Where? No one knows, but we can imagine the crackle of electricity and the blue sparks of neurons firing as a memory is pushed underground, into the furthest and most inaccessible corners of consciousness. There it stays for years, decades, perhaps forever, isolated and protected in a near-dead, dormant state. Removed from the fever of consciousness, it sleeps. Time passes. And then something happens. Sunlight slices through trees. A black leather belt lies curled up, snakelike, on the floor. A word or a phrase is dropped, or a strange but familiar silence falls. And suddenly the memory rises from the deep, a perfectly preserved entity drifting up from the still waters of a once-frozen pond. What causes the glaciated surface of a mind to melt, permitting a buried memory to emerge into consciousness? Where had the memory been hiding all those years? And how do we know that this resuscitated memory, while it looks real, sounds real, and feels real, is not some contaminated mixture of fact and fiction, dream and imagination, fear and desire?[2]

The notion of repression is based on Sigmund Freud's early theories and techniques and is "the cornerstone on which the whole structure of psychoanalysis rests."[3] His teachings provide a good starting point for our investigation, helping us to understand how and why his disciples practice regressionism today.

There are two phrases you'll want to keep in mind, *repression* and *regression*. While they sound very similar, they actually refer to different processes. Repression is a theory about memory loss that Freud invented during the early part of his career. It maintains that a person who experiences a traumatic event can have a complete absence of awareness or memory of that trauma from the time of its occurrence until years, decades, or even centuries later. Meanwhile, regression (and regressionism) refers to a worldview and a collection of memory enhancement techniques that therapists promote as capable of unlocking hidden memories. Repression is a theory about how memories are lost, while regression involves theories on how memories are recovered.

In the late 1800s Freud experimented with eighteen patients who had been diagnosed with *hysteria*. Hysteria, at the time, was characterized by medical symptoms and emotional outbursts for which there were no known physical explanations. Freud suspected that hysteria was not a physical disease at all but rather evidence of repressed memories of sexual abuse. These memories were too painful to tolerate and were therefore "repressed" into the unconscious. Freud explained, "At the bottom of every case of hysteria there are one or more occurrences of premature sexual experience, occurrences which belong to the earliest years of childhood but which can be reproduced through the work of psychoanalysis in spite of the intervening decades."[4]

Repressing painful memories was seen as a psychological defense, an intentional and deliberate method of psychological coping and self-preservation. In order to eliminate hysteria, Freud believed he needed to find a patient's repressed memories and help him have a *cathartic release* or *abreaction*, that is, to become consciously aware of hidden trauma and to express the painful emotions that had been locked away so long. This was achieved through the use of hypnosis, which Freud believed was an essential step in the patient's healing. It was only after these steps that unconscious sources of dysfunctional behaviors could be relieved That, as his theory goes, would cure the patient's hysteria.

The Descent of Psychology

Once you have the cap and gown all you need do is
open your mouth.
Whatever nonsense you talk becomes wisdom and all
the rubbish, good sense.
MOLIÈRE, *THE IMAGINARY INVALID*, 1673

Psychology, the study of human thought and behavior, has actually existed for approximately 2,500 years in various philosophies and theologies. But in the late nineteenth century psychology was reborn as a scientific discipline that sought to use proposed theories, carefully controlled experiments, and statistical analysis to advance our knowledge about human behaviors and potential psychological treatments.

But psychology has changed dramatically since its rebirth. Over 350 "denominations" of psychotherapy have come about,[5] each with its own school of thought about the nature of man, the goals of therapy, and the best techniques. This has led to a cacophony of wild and enthusiastic claims. It's like being at a flea market and having different vendors shouting out the fantastic benefits of their particular cures and potions. Unfortunately, the degeneration of psychology escalated in the 1960s with the emergence of "pop" psychology, ranging from primal scream therapy and sleep-deprivation weekends to acid trips and art expression.

Here's a good example of what I'm talking about. As I'm writing this chapter, I've received a colorful brochure in the mail promoting an upcoming four-day conference for therapists. Here's a sampling of some of the classes offered:

- Embracing Soul, Inviting Spirit: Near-death experiences and other doorways to our soul
- Heart of Peace: a participatory musical event
- The Rubenfeld Synergy Method®: healing the emotional and spiritual body
- Equine (Horse) Therapy: healing ourselves with animals
- On the Other Hand: engaging the wisdom of your other hand
- The Alexander Technique: the gentle elegance of posture and touch
- The Soul Echo of Hawaii: the call to the heart
- The Living Genogram: awakening the families within us
- The Body as Storyteller: wisdom and guidance from the language of the body
- Phoenix Rising Yoga Therapy: using the body as a doorway to the soul
- The Music of Deep Space: returning to the stars
- Night Writer: exploring your dreams through journaling
- The Tooth Fairy, Easter Bunny, Santa, and God: using music and humor to get unstuck![6]

Therapists are invited to join colleagues for four days of training at a plush resort. And better yet, participants will receive valuable continuing education credits from a host of national counselor accreditation programs.

It would be nice to say that this kind of conference is a rare exception, but that is not the case. Unfortunately, a large segment of psychology has degenerated into social, political, and New Age advocacy groups that have made psychology a breeding ground for the most fantastic and irresponsible theories and practices. Activists have made effective use of creative statistics, psychobabble, and unproved theories in lending an air of pseudoscientific respectability to their various agendas. Having abandoned critical reasoning and science in favor of social change and "feel good" theories, psychology has become, for many, less of a forum for the scientific pursuit of truth and more of a propaganda tool to usher in a "New World Order."[7]

Disturbingly, techniques that arose from the pop psychology movement were put into practice without formal testing for safety and validity. In contrast, other professions have developed independent review boards that protect consumers from dangerous practices. For instance, the Food and Drug Administration carefully tests and monitors medications to ensure that a product does what it claims and harmful side effects are accounted for. Such is not the case in psychology, which has increasingly accepted nontested and faddish treatment methods, much to the detriment of society. It was in this setting that a resurrection of Freud's theory of repression took hold of the psychological community.

Different Forms of Repression

Simple repression is what Freud originally had in mind and is said to occur when a patient represses only a handful of traumatic events. But modern regressionists now maintain that *robust repression* also occurs on a regular basis. This is a dramatic extension of repression theory and maintains that volumes of abuse over decades or centuries can be repressed and later recovered. For instance, robust repression is involved in trauma from previous lives, with the idea that literally lifetimes of memories are stored in the unconscious.

Another popular form of robust repression is *multiple-personality disorder (MPD)*.[8] In cases of MPD, regressionists believe that not only are dozens or hundreds of traumatic events repressed, but that separate personalities are developed within the person to "split off" traumatic memories. The theory teaches that a person can have anywhere from two to hundreds of separate personalities living inside him or her, without the person having a knowledge of their existence. These personalities are called *alters* (for "alternate personalities") and take the form of men, women, boys, girls, homosexuals, animals, and demons. They vary in temperament; some are raging, hostile, and focused on mutilating and killing the self, while others are timid and powerless. With time each personality can be coaxed into sharing the "memories" it alone possesses, and with years of expensive therapy it is believed that dozens of the personalities can be reintegrated into a happy, harmonic whole within the person. But all is not as its proponents would have it seem. The existence of an actual MPD disorder is hotly disputed in psychology and to date there is no scientific evidence that the traumatic events reported by many MPDs are actual, historical events.

Strange Bedfellows

So who are the people that promote regressionism? On a national level there are four social groups: *feminists, Christians, New Agers,* and *Science-fiction advocates.* In my work with regressionists, I've noticed that the different regression camps (much like competing denominations) tend to not get along with each other. Each group is certain that it's the real thing while the other "denominations" are ruining credibility for actual victims. Feminists assert their hypnotic images are authentic and wish the space alien advocates would quit making their outrageous claims. Meanwhile, ritual abuse believers are often Christians who side with the feminists, but take offense at the stories of the New Agers who journey into past lives. The New Agers, who side with the space alien advocates, are disgusted by the Christians who are so closed-minded. In last place, the space alien advocates get the least respect and just want to be invited to the party.

As I've talked with regressionists from the different "denominations," I've found they take great offense at being associated with the "others." Usually they'll ask me to quit bringing up the other denominations and stick with their particular camp (which is, of course, the legitimate one). Interestingly, when I ask one camp about other forms of repressed memories, they explain them according to their own particular worldview. The feminists tell me that recovered memories of space alien traumas are due to an abused child's distortion of actual sexual abuse. The Christian regressionists agree with the feminists but point out that space alien abductions are actually satanic ritual abuses in which the victim has been preprogrammed to see the cult members as space aliens. Meanwhile, the Science-fiction advocates tell me that ritual-abuse believers are actually seeing traumas on spaceships but because of religious bias are mistaking the images as being satanic in nature. The New Age believers agree with the Science-fiction advocates and feminists, but think that the Christians are misguided fanatics and that satanic ritual abuse (SRA) is actually space alien and past life trauma that has been distorted.

Of particular interest to me is the fact that a regression believer *never* tells me that the other denominations are having false memories. Contrary memories are always explained as a distortion of a "real abuse event" ("real abuse" being defined by the person I'm talking to). To allow for the possibility of false memories, at any level, is to ultimately endanger one's own denomination—"If it could be false in their case, it could be false in mine." Therefore, the underlying belief in repressed memories is always affirmed, while discrepancies are reshaped into each camp's particular world conspiracy.

The Books

Round about what is, lies a whole mysterious world of might be, a psychological romance of possibilities and things that do not happen.
LONGFELLOW, "TABLE TALK," *DRIFTWOOD*, 1857

Books and articles have played a prominent role in promoting the message of regressionism. Wide-scale interest in repressed memories died down after the turn of the century. But a book on prior lives got the ball rolling again in 1956, when Morey Bernstein released *The Search for Bridey Murphy*.[9] Bernstein, an amateur hypnotist, reported that he had taken his neighbor, Virginia Tighe, back to a previous life in the early 1800s. Though his book was later debunked, Bernstein sparked a national interest in hypnosis and reincarnation. Many popular books promoting past lives and regression techniques have since followed, including *Past Lives Therapy, Recalling Past Lives, Life Before Life, You Have Been Here Before, Past Lives, Future Lives, Blame It on Your Past Lives*, and *Dancing in the Light*.

Multiple-Personality and Satanic Ritual Abuse

An early promotion of multiple-personality disorder (MPD) and abuses in childhood was *The Three Faces of Eve*, an account of one woman's ordeal. In its footsteps came *Michelle Remembers*, in which Michelle Smith claims that she had MPD and recounted her recovered memories of being in a satanic cult where cult members tore apart live kittens, cut fetuses in half, raped her with a crucifix, and forced her to defecate on the Bible. During her therapy sessions, Michelle would develop "body memories" which included the mark of Satan's tail wrapping around her neck. Other popular SRA and MPD books followed, including *Sybil*, *Breaking the Circle of Satanic Ritual Abuse*, and *Uncovering the Mystery of MPD*.

Space Alien Abductions

Since the 1980s another popular series of books has reported the "tragedy" of millions of space alien abductions. Popular titles have included *Communion: A True Story*, *Aliens Among Us*, and *Out There*. Typically the victims cannot remember their abductions, but they have strange symptoms and flashbacks that point the way to a horrible, buried secret. Finally, under self- or therapist-induced hypnosis the victim is able to see his or her space alien traumas.

Forgotten Sexual Abuse

There are numerous books promoting regressionism, but by far the most popular has been *The Courage to Heal*. Written by two authors with no formal degrees in psychology, the book promotes exotic regression theories, lesbian lifestyles, and the need to sustain and nurture one's hatred and anger against parents. Amazingly, the majority of *Christian* regressionists I've talked to regularly recommend this book to their clients. Some quotes from this book include:

> If you are unable to remember any specific instances [of abuse] but still have a feeling that something abusive happened to you, it probably did.[10]

> So far, no one we've talked to thought she might have been abused, and then later discovered that she hadn't been. The progression always goes the other way, from suspicion to confirmation. If you think you were abused and your life shows the symptoms, then you were.[11]

If you don't remember your abuse, you are not alone. Many women don't have memories, and some never get memories. This doesn't mean they weren't abused.[12]

[In a section offering advice to counselors] You must believe that your client was sexually abused, even if she sometimes doubts it herself. . . . If a client is unsure that she was abused but thinks she might have been, work as though she was.[13]

Other popular titles promoting repressed sexual abuse have included *Secret Survivors*, *Repressed Memories*, *Trauma and Recovery*, and *Victims No Longer: Men Recovering from Incest and Other Sexual Child Abuse*.

Common Themes

Although each repression denomination has its own authoritative works, there are common themes to be found among the different books. These include:

Compelling stories. Each book discusses highly emotional and detailed stories that victims recovered after decades or centuries of forgetting. The stories typically lack independent, verified evidence, but they are told in a highly convincing fashion and are backed by unconfirmed sources.

Teaching repression as fact. With impressive-sounding, elaborate theories, the notion of repression is taught as fact and statements by "experts" are presented. Faulty research studies are cited and phantom statistics are discussed in an effort to lend an air of credibility. (We'll review some of these in Chapter 3.)

Epidemic proportions of abuse. People forgetting incest, survivors of satanic ritual abuse, space alien abductions, and hurts in prior lives are always shown to be in the millions! This suggests there is a raging epidemic that is destroying unsuspecting victims throughout the world and it is only now that we are coming to terms with the crisis.

Special symptoms. There is always a special group of symptoms that indicates the reader has forgotten his or her trauma. By recognizing the signs, readers can follow the trail back to their forgotten abuse. (We'll take a closer look at these lists in Chapter 6.)

Conspiracy theories. There is always an excuse as to why there is no direct evidence related to actual cases of repression. In fact, lack of evidence is proof of whichever trauma is being promoted. If it weren't for the suppressive white males, evil, multigenerational satanists, government cover-up, or closed-minded Christians, the evidence would come to light and the entire world would know the truth that the regressionists have already uncovered.

Regression therapy as a pathway to healing. Each book reveals that there is hope! If the reader applies the techniques of regressionism, he or she too will be able to unlock forgotten traumas. Typically taught are variations on how to self-induce into a hypnotic trance (without any of the warnings we'll explore in Chapter 8). No proof of crimes is needed. No waiting in line. Just stake your claim and join the victims' club.

How Does Someone Come Up with Repressed Images?

In 1895, Freud described how he helped patients produce their repressed images of abuse:

The behavior of patients while they are reproducing these infantile experiences is in every respect incompatible with the assumption that the scenes are anything else than a reality which is being felt with distress and reproduced with the greatest reluctance. Before they come for analysis the patients know nothing about these scenes. They are indignant as a rule if we warn them that such scenes are going to emerge. Only the strongest compulsion of the treatment can induce them to embark on a reproduction of them. While they are recalling these infantile experiences to consciousness, they suffer under the most violent sensations, of which they are ashamed and which they try to conceal; and, even after they have gone through them once more in such a convincing manner, they still attempt to withhold belief from them, by emphasizing the fact that, unlike what happens in the case of other forgotten material, they have no feeling of remembering the scenes.[14]

From the very inception of the regression movement, we learn that the hypnotic images have a great deal to do with therapists' expectations. Through hypnotic techniques and manipulation the client is slowly drawn into believing suggested fantasies as real. Regressionists promote a variety of hypnotic techniques, including traditional hypnosis, self-hypnosis, age-regression, body massage, the use of crystals, trance-writing, dream work, spirit guides, "Holy Spirit hypnosis," and sodium amytal interviews. Guided imagery is one of the more popular methods for retrieving memories and was my personal favorite. I would lead a patient into a relaxed state with her eyes closed and have her imagine getting progressively younger until she reached her early childhood. Then I would have her search for hidden memories I believed were locked inside her. Sure enough, the memories would spill forth.

Sandra is a typical regressionist. She declares that the majority of her clients have been abused in some way, most of them sexually. Some have always remembered their abuse, but others only come to remember with the aid of therapy methods that range from guided imagery sessions to more adventurous art therapy. Sandra adds a novel aspect—she asks the client to imagine being in a childhood home. "As they're doing this, they might describe how they are feeling. They may move into some rooms, and I'll ask 'Who's in these rooms? What are they doing?' And then the memories come."[15]

Sandra regularly regresses clients back into the womb, helping them to relive harmful things said about them and memories of their birth. She also believes repressed memories of abuse can be accessed through art. When clients cannot find the root of their problems, she often asks them to express their feelings through drawings or dance.

> Often what happens is somebody will be moving like they're pushing away, and at a certain point—this almost always happens—they will have images of who they're pushing away. . . . They'll be pushing away their brother or grandfather, mother, father, neighbor, whoever it was who was the perpetrator. And they can begin saying "No" or "Stop" or "Get away" when they weren't able to do that in the original experience because they were overpowered by that person.[16]

Like most therapists, Sandra is a disciple of the popular sixties' notion that "Truth is relative." "I don't know if that's real memory. . . . It's what they imagine it to be, but I don't know if it's really what it was." But she concludes, "I don't care if the details are true or not. What matters is that a person is accessing whatever is true for them in that moment. If it's not the exact experience, so what? What's important is that they have pain around it and want to heal it."[17]

Sandra is firm in her conviction that her clients are not simply imagining the memories they recover. They reflect an underlying truth that the client must be encouraged to access. She is not alone in her beliefs. Nationally, more than a quarter of therapists believe that, "I trust my client such that if he or she says something happened, it must have happened, regardless of the age or context in which the event occurred."[18] Thirty-six percent agree: "If a client believes a memory is true, I must also believe it to be true if I am to help him or her."[19]

Induction into Regressionism

The truth of these days is not that which really is, but what every man persuades another man to believe.
MONTAIGNE, "ON GIVING THE LIE," *ESSAYS*, 1580-88

Usually my clients didn't begin their therapy with regression in mind. Typically they started therapy because of some kind of problem in their lives (depression, marriage problems, poor self-esteem). Regressionists use a sequence of steps in developing recovered images of abuse in a client. Within the first few sessions they read off a list of "indicators" of forgotten abuse. These symptoms lists are a key agent in establishing a belief in the client that "something" is hidden inside of them.

After this initial stage the use of various hypnotic techniques is introduced. The techniques go by a number of names, but each involves the same process for creating a deeply relaxed state in which a client is vulnerable to suggestion and is able to imagine vividly. (We'll discuss different forms of hypnosis in a moment.) While under the influence of these techniques the client starts to experience detailed fantasies of traumatic events and have similar dreams at night. Then, in contradiction to what is known about hypnotic trance and dream states, the client is told that these images are "flashbacks" of real events.

As the patients begin to have more flashbacks of trauma, they begin to decompensate, that is, their personality and ability to function deteriorate dramatically. As their decompensation increases, they are told that their psychotic breakdown is proof that what they fantasized is real. They become increasingly vulnerable to suggestions with each hypnotherapy session and begin to isolate from family and friends who do not support these newfound revelations. As the patient becomes increasingly alienated, she has only the regression leader and group members to turn to, leading to deeper belief and dependency.

Forms of Hypnosis

Regressionists promote a variety of hypnotic techniques in order to induce a relaxed, altered state of mind in a client, including traditional hypnosis, self-hypnosis, age-regression, trance-writing, body massage, the use of crystals, dream work, guided imagery, the use of spirit guides, "Holy Ghost Hypnosis," and sodium amytal interviews. Here is a brief explanation of each:

In traditional **hypnosis** a person is instructed to close her eyes and get into a relaxed, comfortable position. In a soft, monotone voice the hypnotist guides a client into deeper levels of relaxation and begins to make suggestions or ask questions. The client focuses on a mental image while becoming less aware of her physical surroundings.

This same process can be taught to the client for purposes of **self-hypnosis.** In a self-induced trance state the client is able to create vivid fantasies apart from being in the actual presence of her therapist. A portion of the population (referred to as Fantasy Prone Personalities and Grade Fives, discussed in Chapter 10) are naturally self-trancing and regularly do so without any formal training. Many regression believers have told me they received their traumatic fantasies away from the presence of their therapist, therefore their images must be real. But the reality is, they've simply engaged in self-hypnosis. Whether therapist- or self-induced, all the limitations of trance state still apply, which we'll discuss in Chapter 8.

When experiencing **age regression,** a hypnotized client is told a metaphor, such as boarding a train that is going backwards or lying down on a cloud that is moving back in time. The imagery moves the person back into younger time periods and events. This is one of the more popular techniques used in regressionism and was my personal favorite.

In **trance-writing** a client is hypnotized and then given a pad and paper and instructed to allow her "inner child" to draw and express hidden memories and feelings. Often the client is told to use her non-dominant hand, because this "taps into her unconscious processes."

Body massage involves bringing the person into a very relaxed state through physical massage. During this process, the regressionist verbally coaches the client, while seeking to locate places in the body where cells have stored the memory of a particular trauma. It is believed that massaging this group of cells allows the "memories" to be released, freeing them to travel back up to the brain to be remembered. In a similar fashion, **crystals** are sometimes rubbed on different parts of the body, allowing "memories" locked in body parts to be released.

Dream work involves a client being hypnotized and then re-experiencing a dream they've recently had. With the regressionist's guidance, the client is able to clarify the dream and better identify perpetrators and hidden meanings.

In **guided imagery** a person is hypnotized and then mentally taken to a time or place where they can reexperience a traumatic event, or go somewhere very safe and inviting, like a beach or mountain hideaway.

Spirit Guides are popular with New Age and Christian regressionists. A client is hypnotized and then instructed to walk on a path. Eventually they encounter a very wise person on the path who reveals hidden "truths" to the client. This same technique renamed as **"Holy Spirit guidance"** is used by Christian regressionists, who have clients encounter "Jesus" who leads them through the past.

Sodium amytal is a barbiturate drug that produces a physical state of deep relaxation. Once administered, the client enters into a drug-altered state and is asked questions by the regressionist. The client is usually misled in believing that this is a "truth serum" in which they cannot lie.

Freud's Betrayal of the Regressionists

Early in his career, Freud believed that the hypnotic fantasies his patients were describing were real events, and he came out publicly to express his concern that horrible things were happening to children. But as he continued in his research, Freud began to question the reality of his patients' recovered memories. Through his clinical work he became increasingly convinced of unconscious sexual factors shaping his clients' reports of suddenly remembered abuse.

The turning point came on September 21, 1897, when Freud wrote his now-famous letter to his colleague, Dr. Fleiss. "I will confide in you at once the great secret that has been slowly dawning on me in the last few months. I no longer believe in my neurotica [theory of the neuroses]."[20] He became convinced that his hysterics' accounts of abuse, which he had believed to be true, were in fact fantasies. Freud had reached this conclusion as he noticed that his hysterics weren't being cured and that they were developing increasingly vivid and shocking fantasies during hypnosis, which they believed to be true. Freud eventually developed the concept of *psychical reality*, which states that a person can experience a trauma in his or her mind that feels very real but is in fact pure fantasy. Freud concluded that fantasies of abuse reflected underlying conflicts within the unconscious mind.

In an act of tremendous courage, Freud expanded on his original theory to expose what he thought was the complete story. Interestingly, the practices of today's regressionists are based upon Freud's early ideas, while they completely reject his later work. I've heard various theories offered by regressionists to explain why Freud repudiated his first assertions: "Perhaps Freud was overwhelmed and unable to accept the vast quantity of childhood sexual abuse which he found. Perhaps he was coerced or intimidated by his peers into backing away from his early thinking. Perhaps Freud himself was sexually abused, and his later years were due to his 'denial.'"

Claims such as these don't hold up to an actual examination of his research. From the very beginning Freud had questions about the validity of his patients' reports. It was only with extended research that he was able to confirm his earlier concerns. Regarding his new conclusions, Freud declared, "I must recognize them as the result of honest and forcible intellectual work and must be proud that after going so deep I am still capable of such criticism. Can it be that this doubt merely represents an episode in advance towards further knowledge?"[21]

Was Freud in denial? Did he back down because of pressure from others? No, the fact is that Freud was simply reporting the truth, a truth that science is rediscovering today. But regressionists view Freud as having committed the ultimate betrayal. While they acknowledge him for the contributions that form the entire basis for their movement, they also denounce him for what they interpret to be the eventual "selling out" of their cause. Almost one hundred years later, they still aren't listening to the second half of his findings. In a culture that promotes victim identity, one can see how Freud has been forbidden to voice the rest of the story.

Points to Remember

✓ *Repression* is a theory about memory loss that Freud invented and later rejected. It maintains that a person who experiences a traumatic event can have a complete absence of awareness or memory of that trauma from the time of its occurrence until years, decades, or even centuries later.

✓ *Regression* refers to a number of hypnotic techniques that therapists promote as unlocking hidden memories.

✓ *Simple repression* is said to occur when a patient represses a handful of traumatic events. *Robust repression* expresses the idea that volumes of abuse over decades or centuries can be repressed and later recovered.

✓ Social groups that promote regressionism include feminists, Christians, New Agers, and science-fiction advocates.

✓ Regression literature plays a seminal role in developing a belief system in vulnerable clients. Once that belief system is in place, various hypnotic techniques are used to create vivid fantasies in clients.

✓ After experiencing the hypnotic images, the client typically suffers severe decompensation—his or her personality and ability to function deteriorate dramatically. Each regression session leads to greater vulnerability and dependency on the client's part, and he or she begins to isolate from family and friends who do not support the newfound revelations.

3

Repression Takes the Stand

The great masses of the people . . . will more easily fall victims to a big lie than to a small one.

ADOLPH HITLER, *MEIN KAMPF*, 1924

June recalls the phone call that exploded into their lives. Her daughter's voice was clear and distant. Greta quickly got to the point and declared, "Mom, I've figured out what has been making me sick all these years."

June answered, "That's great, honey, what is it?"

"I remember being sexually abused as a child," Greta stated.

"I can't believe it! Who did it?" June exclaimed.

Greta said, "It was Dad."[1]

Greta's "happy childhood" had melted away when she learned in therapy that her depression and tendency to wake up at night with a sensation of being choked were symptoms of repressed memories of sexual abuse. "I went into my bedroom and lay on my bed, and suddenly I felt hands around my throat, choking me. And then I felt myself being pushed under water. I knew I was still in bed, but I felt the whole thing. I felt myself breathe water, and then I went black. I woke up lying in my bed."[2]

From this rather simple memory, the stories became increasingly detailed and gory. One by one each of her sisters got into recovered memory therapy, and soon all five daughters fantasized horrifying details of brutal sexual and psychological abuse by their father, as well as details of murders they had "witnessed" him committing. The accusations snowballed, each more horrible than the last. Their father Roy, former head of the department of engineering at a large state university, was accused by one daughter of repeatedly raping her throughout her childhood, once breaking her cat's neck, and rubbing her body with the corpse. This daughter also says her father tied her to the bumper of his truck and dragged her along a dirt road through a desert mountain park. When he stopped, she claims he dug a grave, partially buried her in it, and left her there for six to eight hours, until he returned to rape her again. Another daughter, who says that the sexual assaults began when she was five years old and continued until she was thirty-three, has even more gruesome "memories." On various occasions, she stated in the lawsuit against her parents that her father forced her to eat feces, nailed her into a wooden crate, and allowed her to be drugged, raped, and *scalped* by his friends. This daughter was able to perform successfully through a typical upper-middle-class lifestyle, even completing medical school, but didn't know about her trauma until she was in therapy.

All five daughters refuse to question their hypnotic images. When two were asked by a newspaper reporter if they could be imagining their abuse, they looked at each other and giggled. Kristi declared, "There just isn't any question about it. If I am sitting here, if this table exists, then I was abused."[3] The sisters maintain that a brother was an active observer during one of the murders, but he has no such memories. He told the same reporter in a phone interview, "I don't have any memory of anything like my sisters are talking about, there wasn't anything like that going on."[4] He supposedly was riding with his father when Roy pulled out a .22-caliber gun and randomly shot a young girl riding her bicycle down a road. Years ago a man had confessed to the crime and was sentenced to life in prison. But Maria, another one of the daughters, still holds firm to her story. They also have accused Roy of murdering several other women, although the facts surrounding the cases disprove any possible involvement on his part.

The daughters tried to sue their father based on their fantasies of abuse. But their case quickly fell apart under initial investigation, and the legal proceedings were quickly dropped. It is small comfort for June and Roy, who have lost five beloved daughters to regressionism. "We know the girls believe what they have said, but if they could just begin to question it a little bit. . . ."[5]

The Search for Truth

C. S. Lewis, in referring to the Christian faith, describes the need to examine its claims:

> Here is the door, behind which, according to some people, the secret of the universe is waiting for you. Either that's true, or it isn't. And if it isn't, then what the door really conceals is simply

the greatest fraud, the most colossal "sell" on record. Isn't it obviously the job of every man (that is a man and not a rabbit) to try to find out which, and then to devote his full energies either to serving this tremendous secret or to exposing and destroying this gigantic humbug?[6]

Much like a religious faith, regressionism has become a new gospel for many and promises powerful healing to its faithful disciples. When I entered the world of regressionism I was convinced that I had found a golden key to unlock hidden truths, a marvelous discovery which held incredible potential. I believed, and taught, that what I was doing was the latest in scientific techniques.

Brian Weiss, the Harvard psychiatrist and best-selling author I mentioned in chapter 1, is nationally known for his work with taking clients back in time to previous lives. He sees himself as the next Galileo, who was persecuted by the church in the seventeenth century for claiming that the earth was not the center of the solar system.

The scientists of his day would not even look through his telescope. . . . After all, it was a tool of the devil. . . . We're just saying "Look, here's another telescope and this is what I'm seeing; won't you take a look and tell me what you see?" That's science. It's not having your mind made up before you look.[7]

That said, the American Psychiatric Association is less than enthusiastic: "Past-life regression is pure quackery. As in other areas of medicine, psychiatric diagnosis and treatment today is based on objective scientific evidence. There is no accepted scientific evidence to support the existence of past lives, let alone the validity of past-life regression therapy."[8]

Dr. Weiss takes umbrage with this criticism. So let's stop a moment to ask: Is regressionism the new science? Are those who question regressionists' bold claims members of the "Flat Earth Society"? As we examine the evidence to support regressionism, it is important to understand basic aspects of scientific research.

Science deals with *confirmable propositions* that can be confirmed or falsified *publicly*—any researcher should be capable of replicating an experiment and get the same results. Notice that science is not concerned with private or unique events that cannot be proved. The statement, "When I eat five tomatoes a day I am more relaxed at work," is scientifically useless because it refers to a personal experience that is unique and undemonstratable. However, the statement, "People who eat five tomatoes a day tend to be more relaxed," is scientific because it is verifiable—it can be proved true or false. A researcher could have a group of subjects eat five tomatoes a day, another group that doesn't, and then compare their anxiety levels on an objective test for stress. If researchers can repeat the procedure enough times with the same results, they have discovered a *scientific law*—a consistent relationship between two or more events. If there is no way to publicly demonstrate a statement or theory as true or false, it is scientifically worthless.

Science maintains a healthy skepticism, and those who promote a new theory are required to present evidence to back it up. *Theories* are developed to explain things that we observe in nature, and they set the stage for scientific verification. Often a theory can sound really good but be completely false. There is always a danger of being overly impressed by its wording and overlooking the fact that there is no demonstrable evidence for what it predicts. For example, astrology is a highly developed theory, but it has little or no demonstrated validity. In other words, it *sounds* good, but its claims don't stand up under scientific investigation.

Empirical evidence involves objective findings that can be verified by anyone. *Anecdotal evidence* is made up of stories that are based on personal experience. The problem with anecdotal evidence is that it is difficult and often impossible to verify. Anecdotal claims can be very important for exploratory research, but it is imperative that the case for a theory be founded in empirical evidence. This allows scientists to objectively determine the reality of a phenomenon, while avoiding getting pulled into "faddish" or superstitious claims.

Before I bore you too much, understand this has direct relevance to the repression theories. One of the first things I learned in my training to recover memories is that there are theories that explain everything. Using technical terms that sounded authoritative, I was taught lots of theories about how traumatic memory is different than normal memory, how the body can store memories in the cells of different body parts, *ad infinitum*. But these theories are not to be confused with providing actual evidence. So is there scientific evidence for repression? Let's look at three of the most commonly cited studies.

The Scientific Case for Repression

Herman and Schatzow

In 1987 two therapists worked with fifty-three women in a twelve-week incest survivors group. They claimed that 74 percent of the women were able to validate their memories of abuse by obtaining corroborating evidence. But there are several problems with their study. First, most of these subjects (72 percent) had full or partial recall of their abuse (free-standing memories). Remember our discussion in Chapter 1? The false memory controversy does not include free-standing memories. So to begin with, nearly all of the subjects' abuse had nothing to do with repressed memories.

Second, details of corroboration were vague and depended upon self-report, without independent confirmation. The researchers describe their group of subjects as histrionic, borderline, avoidant, depressed, anxiety prone, and suicidal. Confirming evidence deemed acceptable was a box of dirty magazines, a set of handcuffs found at home, and other such inconclusive items. It is very important to understand that there was absolutely *no* independent corroboration for these mentally disturbed subjects' reports.[9]

Far from demonstrating repression, this study confirmed that two therapists were able to collect uncorroborated evidence of abuse from mentally unstable subjects who were given a twelve-week assignment to prove abuse and were then rewarded in therapy. This study is seriously flawed and for the most part doesn't deal with repressed memories. I initially believed the study's statistics. It was only as I later read the actual study that I realized it was simply not true.

One of the researchers, Dr. Herman buys into the idea of "relative truth." She admits that the evidence her subjects produced probably would fall short of convincing a jury, but she's not particularly concerned about the accuracy of hypnotic images.

> If an adult wants to say "I have come to understand my life in a certain way that makes sense to me, a way that helps me live my life and make sense of my symptoms," then that's something an adult is entitled to do. . . . Sometimes they're just looking for a smoking gun to make [their troubles] look serious enough. Since they are not used to having their wishes or needs taken seriously, sometimes people will only feel validated in a certain sense if they are able to put that kind of a name [abuse] on it.[10]

One wonders if this would be the same standard she would apply if a client sued her for mental health fraud. "Well, your honor," she might say, "my former client wants me to pay her ten million dollars, to have my license revoked, and to have me spend a few years in jail. I would have to agree. She's an adult who doesn't need to produce any proof of her charges. She's made sense out of her symptoms, and she should have her wishes and needs validated."

"Barbara," a Christian grandmother, has been accused by her thirty-one-year-old daughter of being a murdering, satanic high priestess. She comments on Herman's rationalizations: "You're allowing these people to build their egos and self-esteem on lies. What Ms. Herman is saying is that honesty and reality mean absolutely nothing in therapy today."[11] The fact is, truth matters, regardless of Herman's firm assertions to the contrary.

Briere and Conte

In a second study, researchers John Briere and Jon Conte interviewed 468 people who had reported a history of sexual abuse. In all, 59.6 percent of those questioned indicated that at some time they had forgotten their abuse. Only one question was asked about repression. It is stated here, verbatim, complete with the errors in grammar that appeared in their questionnaire:

"During the period of time before the first forced sexual experienced happened and your eighteenth birthday was there ever a time when you could not remember the forced sexual experience?"[12]

What are the problems with this study? First, the question is confusing—it means different things to different people. Second, like the previous study, it is purely anecdotal, with no independent confirmation of the described abuse. Most importantly, the study uses a classic form of circular reasoning. A subject was identified as being a victim of abuse because she had hypnotic images of abuse. But how do we know that the images are real? Because she is a victim of abuse. This is the same technique used for space alien abductions: "We know that this person was abducted by aliens because he repressed the trauma. He repressed the trauma because the aliens forced it from his mind," or "She was tortured by the satanic cult, and they hypnotized her into forgetting all the trauma. We know this is true because she now has recovered memories of them doing these things." What we know from this study is that 60 percent of people responding to a poorly worded questionnaire claim that they were abused because they have had traumatic hypnotic images. It is just as likely an indicator of the extent of false memories as it is evidence for repression.

Williams

In 1992, Linda Williams attempted a more scientific study. She interviewed more than one hundred women who were victims of childhood sexual abuse in the mid-1970s. These cases had been recorded in police files, which allowed for independent confirmation of their abuse. Seventeen years later, Williams and her colleagues interviewed the women to see if they would report the original abuse without directly being asked about it. It was found that 38 percent of the women did not reveal their abuse to the interviewer.[13]

In a similar study done several years *earlier*, Donna Femina and fellow researchers interviewed subjects with documented histories of physical abuse. Precisely 38 percent also gave a history that did not reveal documented abuse. But Femina and her colleagues went back and found eleven of those subjects for a follow-up interview. They asked them why they hadn't revealed their abuse. Each acknowledged they remembered but simply had chosen not to reveal the events because of embarrassment, a desire to protect parents, or a desire to forget.[14]

Femina's study is by no means unique. A number of studies have demonstrated what scientists call *failure to disclose*, a reluctance on the part of subjects to disclose embarrassing information to researchers. Think about it—common sense tells us that a person isn't likely to tell a complete stranger about the time a family member sodomized her. Would you?

And this is the problem with Williams' study—she simply didn't go on to the next step as Femina did. It is impossible to determine if her subjects truly forgot their abuse or simply chose not to tell strangers about such deeply personal traumas. But even if some did forget, it still does not point to a repression phenomenon. As we shall see in the next chapter, forgetting and repressing are actually two different concepts. Many of the subjects, toddlers at the time of the abuse, were simply too young to encode the abuse into long-term memory storage. Another interesting side note: Williams' extensive reference section fails to acknowledge Femina's published study, one that is exactly on point to her own and easily found through a standard search of the literature. Now this was either due to negligence on Williams' part or was by design. Either way, it raises serious concerns about the integrity of her study.

All three of these studies have serious flaws that leave them outside the realm of serious scientific research. A recent landmark court decision, *State of New Hampshire v. Joel Hungerford*, has declared repression to be scientifically unreliable. In commenting on the research evidence, the court came to the following conclusions:

> Several recent survey studies have been cited to support the existence of the phenomenon of repressed memories for traumatic events. . . . Many of these were survey studies, not clinical studies. Attempts to interpret the results of these studies as evidence of the existence of repressed memory are severely restricted because of certain methodological and other deficiencies inherent in the studies. Many of the studies failed to adequately account for so-called childhood amnesia, that is, the recognized inability or reduced ability of children to form narrative memories before the age of 5. Few of the studies confirm or corroborate the occurrence of the alleged trauma in any way. . . . In many of the survey studies . . . the survey question was sufficiently ambiguous, that it is not possible to ascertain whether the failure to remember the experience was in fact memory repression, or merely normal forgetting or reluctance to disclose the event. . . . Even the highly regarded study by Linda Meyer Williams in 1994, which did confirm the occurrence of the traumatic event, exhibits serious methodological deficiencies which impair the validity of its results. Specifically, the lack of a follow-up interview undermines confidence in the study's conclusion of the existence of repressed memory. The failure to report abuse could have resulted from reluctance to disclose, ordinary forgetting or a myriad of other factors. Furthermore, the influence of childhood amnesia in the Williams study was not sufficiently considered. These methodological deficiencies in these recent studies have caused the field of psychology to approach the concept of repressed memory with some skepticism.[15]

The Scientific Case Against Repression

Some circumstantial evidence is very strong,
as when you find a trout in the milk.
THOREAU, *JOURNAL*, 1850

Lori was a woman with a horrifying secret. At the age of five, she saw her father savagely strike her mother, and later that night heard him digging in the backyard. Her mother was never seen again, and it was assumed that she had run away to get out of a troubled marriage. But Lori knew better. The next year a mysterious fire occurred in the home while her father was out running an errand. An older sister threw herself on Lori to protect her from the flames. Lori survived with burns over 50 percent of her body, but both of her older sisters died. For twenty-eight years she kept her dark secrets, terrified that her father would try to kill her as well. Finally, she wrote a letter to the police because she couldn't live with her memories. "In spite of my fears, I decided that I'd rather be dead than to keep the secret."[16] Police found her mother's remains buried in the backyard of the family's home.

Based on the theory of repression, Lori, alone and threatened for her life, should have repressed the horrific events that had happened to herself and family members. But throughout the years she has been able to freely recall these horrors, without the aid of hypnosis or other regression techniques. In the subsequent trial, one attorney noted that Lori's free-standing memories made her a more credible witness: "I don't think the general public finds 'repressed memories' credible."[17]

And herein lies the regressionists' greatest dilemma: Their theories don't work in the real world. When we know that a traumatic event has occurred, we find that victims don't repress their traumatic experiences. Instead they are plagued by recurring memories of their trauma, sometimes resulting in *post-traumatic stress disorder* (discussed in the next chapter).

A recent study was done on preschoolers who have experienced serious trauma resulting in a visit to the emergency room. They were interviewed immediately after their accidents, six months later, and finally, one year later. In not one instance did a child repress their trauma. It was also found that their level of stress didn't have an interfering effect on remembering. At the one year interval, it was found they experienced normal aspects of forgetting, but none had forgotten the entire event.[18]

Other studies that have tracked bona fide victims of trauma yield predictable results, a few of which bear mentioning.

- One study found that children who had witnessed the murder of a parent didn't repress their memories; rather, they were preoccupied with the murders and they were continually flooded with disturbing emotions.[19]

- Of the dozens of children kidnapped in Chowchilla, California in 1976, none were found to have repressed their memories of the event.[20]
- Paul McHugh, Director of Psychiatry at Johns Hopkins University Medical School, has worked extensively with Cambodian refugees. Based on the theories of multiple personality we would expect to find some portion of these children having developed MPD. But despite experiencing the horrors of war as children, McHugh has not found one case of repression or multiple-personality disorder (MPD).[21]
- In another study, researchers interviewed seventy-eight Holocaust survivors forty years after the end of World War II. Though each of the people had experienced normal memory decay, none had repressed memories of their prison camp experiences, and all but one quickly remembered forgotten details with simple prompting.[22]

In considering the groups of actual victims noted above, none behaves as repression theory predicts. As was the case with Lori, these victims remember almost everything and repress nothing. The conclusion? People remember, rather than repress, traumatic events. A court ruling supports this finding:

Research and studies of memory in general and traumatic memory in particular have indicated that in general, traumatic events are well remembered. However, studies have indicated that some degree of memory disturbance is commonly associated with traumatic experiences. Studies have indicated that hyperamnesia, i.e. intrusive memories of the event, and partial amnesia of parts of the event, are common for those who have experienced a traumatic event. Studies indicate that the gist of the traumatic event is generally extremely well retained, while the details may be inaccurate.[23]

The New Science?

So is repression the new science? Like Dr. Weiss, our past-life promoter, I fervently believed it was and taught my clients about this newly discovered passageway pointing to the boldest frontier of human exploration. The theories I was taught were long-winded and very scholarly sounding. But upon closer examination I found them to have no basis in real science—there simply was no tangible evidence to support these theories as real. For that matter, the evidence was actually contrary to what I was teaching. Dr. David Holmes, an expert in the area of research on memory and repression, noted:

> Despite over sixty years of research involving numerous approaches by many thoughtful and clever investigators, at the present time there is no controlled laboratory evidence supporting the concept of repression. . . . Despite numerous tests [we don't] have data to support the theory, and therefore it might be appropriate to abandon the theory. From a practical standpoint, data provide the "bottom line." They are the test of the theory. If the data have been adequately collected but are inconsistent with what is predicted by the theory, then we must ask serious questions about the theory, elegant as it may be. . . . Regardless of how fascinating the repression hypothesis is, the time may have come to move on.[24]

Dr. Weiss regards those who question the theory of repression as intellectual midgets who refuse to look through the telescope of science. Well, I looked, I saw what was there, and for a time I believed. But then I began to allow myself to look from other perspectives and discover that the evidence simply wasn't there. The fact is, the regressionist's new telescope wasn't holding up to scientific scrutiny.

You may ask, "Dr. Simpson, are you saying there is no such thing as repression?" Actually, I'm not. What I am saying is there is no scientific evidence of its existence. That's an important distinction. To date, the evidence for repression is based on stories that have not been verified by science, law enforcement, or the legal community. Despite these facts, regressionists still propose that there is a psychological defense mechanism that takes traumatic experiences and pushes them down into a hidden part of the brain or other parts of a person's body, and then decades or centuries later releases perfectly preserved memories into the conscious mind. It's an interesting theory and one that I came to believe as true. But as a psychologist who specializes in treating victims of abuse, I can't point to any empirical or scientific evidence for this claim. In fact, the evidence we have is to the contrary. But in scientific terms, I can't tell you that repression never happens. That would be "proving the negative," an impossible task.

The very best anyone can say at this time is that hypnotic images of incest, ritual tortures, alien abductions, and past lives draw from one of three sources: 1) historical events, 2) pure fantasies, or 3) a bizarre mixing of historical and fantasized elements. Apart from independent, external confirmation, there is no proven way to determine the true source of a hypnotic image. A very real possibility is that some cases of repression are genuine and we simply lack the technology or precision at this time to recognize them as such.

Another question might be, "Okay, maybe we can't be certain that a recovered memory is real. But I've been told there are techniques that can safely unlock memories!" The first question about the existence of repression awaits future confirmation. But this next question about memory recovery can be answered with much greater certainty. Remember that repression is a theory about how memories are lost, while regression involves theories on how memories are recovered. It's important to keep this difference in mind as we ask our next question, "Is there a way to safely and accurately unlock memories?" In a word, no! As we will discover in the following chapters, there is no scientific or biblical technique that can safely and accurately unlock "repressed" events. In fact, the hypnotic techniques that are promoted are consistently shown to create highly suggestible, delusional states of mind in which clients have: 1) a decreased ability to accurately recall historical events, 2) increased experiential fantasy, and 3) increased levels of confidence in the accuracy of their recall, even though this is not the case.[25]

I came across a principle of logic: "When it is impossible to determine what is true, it is important to determine what is most probable." This is a process that I refer to as a *caring skepticism*. While there may be actual cases of repression, traumatic fantasies associated with regression therapy, readings, or recovery groups are far less likely to be real. This is particularly true for clients involved with regression therapy, who are noted for their high suggestibility (we'll discuss this in chapter 10).

Looking for the Grain of Truth

In finding resolution to my questions, it was tempting to look for the conservative "grain of truth": "I'm willing to agree that the recovered memories of space aliens and past lives are false; it's the ones about incest that are mostly real." While at first glance this sounds reasonable and has appeal, there's a problem. It's not true. Hypnotic images of incest are not necessarily any more genuine than hypnotic images of space aliens. But they are more *believable*, which makes them more dangerous.

Let me explain. Suppose a man with a bona fide paranoid delusion comes into a psychologist's office. He sits down on her couch and complains that, lately, space aliens are listening to his thoughts through the fillings in his teeth. Part of his solution is that at night he sleeps with tinfoil wrapped around his head, which, he explains, prevents the aliens from being able to control his mind. He's disturbed because he knows that this isn't quite normal, and his wife, understandably, has urged him to seek therapy.

The psychologist is quickly able to make her diagnosis of paranoid delusions and begin a proper course of treatment. But suppose her next client also has a bona fide paranoid delusion, but this one isn't about space aliens. "I used to work for military intelligence," he says. He shows his discharge papers from three years ago. "I got into a bunch of highly classified stuff, and eventually I just had to get out of the 'business.'" He declares that since his discharge, secret government forces have been keeping a close eye on him. Recently, an old buddy has let him know that an order has been put out to have him killed. Now he sleeps at night with a loaded gun, "Just in case." His wife is scared and urged him to seek help.

This time, in making her diagnosis, the psychologist isn't quite sure what to put down. But remember, both men had severe paranoid delusions, but the second one sounded more reasonable. And herein lies the problem. In psychology we know that the more colorful and fantastic a patient's delusions are, the easier it is to identify and treat, both by the therapist and the patient. But the closer a delusion approximates a real scenario, has real elements and sounds "reasonable," the more difficult it is for the therapist or client to recognize it as such. You see, it's easy for us to write off space alien abductions and past-life traumas, because for many of us these are not part of our belief system. But what if someone has a delusion that does fit into our belief system? C. S. Lewis rightly cautions, "Nothing can deceive unless it bears a plausible resemblance to reality."[26]

Loch Ness Therapy

Let me close with an example that might shed some light on my position. There are those who maintain that there is a Loch Ness monster in Scotland. Now, personally I've never seen a Loch Ness monster, nor is there any scientific evidence that one exists, yet I couldn't tell you that it definitely doesn't exist. Maybe it's a leftover dinosaur from a previous age. Who knows? It's not my task to prove to you one way or the other; it's up to Loch Ness believers to make their case and present the evidence for their theory.

But let's imagine that these same Loch Ness believers go one step further and maintain that there are millions of Loch Ness monsters living in lakes, rivers, and backyard pools throughout America. The believers say Loch Ness monsters are terrorizing and eating hundreds of thousands of victims but no one sees them because the monsters hypnotize their witnesses. In fact, there are individuals who have encountered Loch Ness monsters on dozens of occasions and have forgotten each encounter (referred to as "robust" repression). Because of believers' accusations people have been put in jail as Loch Ness accomplices and countless families have been destroyed.

At this point I must introduce the ideas of *volume* and what is most *probable*. One remains open to the possibility of an unproved theory, but as the volume of what is being alleged increases without a concurrent rise in evidence, the probability decreases. This principle is even more important as the damaging consequences of a proposed theory grow more dramatic.

Let's take one final step in our example. Imagine that the believers become licensed, professional Loch Ness experts, who go door-to-door selling "Monster Kits" for twenty thousand dollars apiece. They maintain that this kit will help people become unhypnotized and will also get rid of the Loch Ness monsters that live in their backyard pools. Mind you, the "kit" contains a number of drugs which create delusional states of mind. Sales go better than expected. Loch Ness believers get great media coverage, publish books, open up inpatient treatment centers, and come to be regarded as "experts" on monster traumas. The concept skyrockets into a multibillion-dollar industry.

But there are those who begin to question the New Order. These skeptics are quickly labeled as heretics who are insensitive to the plight of Loch Ness survivors. It is at this point that we must entertain the idea of consumer fraud. It's one thing to consider the possible validity of a proposed theory and await further evidence. It is quite another matter to be selling "cures" based on these unproved theories and using techniques that are known to create delusional states of mind.

So what is my point? Regarding the Loch Ness monster: 1) The Loch Ness Monster is not scientifically proven, but it is theoretically possible; 2) multiple monsters are far less probable; and 3) treatment kits and Loch Ness therapies are fraudulent. Regarding regressionism: 1) Simple repression of trauma is not scientifically proven, but it is theoretically possible; 2) robust and epidemic repression is far less probable; and 3) memory-enhancement techniques and the regression industry constitute mental-health fraud.

Perhaps you think I'm too far-fetched in my example. Regressionists claim each of us has lived dozens of past lives, that there are thousands of victims of satanic ritual abuse, that we can journey back into the fallopian tubes of our mothers, that there are over one hundred million space alien victims, [27] and there are millions throughout the world who don't remember their own sexual abuse. A huge cottage industry has arisen that promotes dangerous, unproved techniques as "pathways to hidden truths." Now, either this is true or something else is going on. "And if it isn't, then what the door really conceals is simply the greatest fraud, the most colossal 'sell' on record. Isn't it obviously the job of every man . . . to try to find out which, and then to devote his full energies either to serving this tremendous secret or to exposing and destroying this gigantic humbug?"[28]

One of the greatest dangers we face is that the theories of repression have entered into the mainstream of society, and for the majority these theories have been assumed to be valid without any evidence being required. Remember, the theory of repression is just that, an early Freudian theory that waits to be proven. The burden of proof is on the regressionists, and as of yet they have not scientifically proven their theories. In contrast, their techniques have conclusively been shown to create delusional states in which clients' ability to accurately recall events is actually diminished.

Points to Remember

✓ *Empirical evidence* involves objective findings that can be verified by anyone. *Anecdotal evidence* includes stories that are based on personal experience.

✓ Despite claims to the contrary, there is still little scientific evidence supporting the concept of repression. Research is consistent in showing that people remember, rather than repress, traumatic events. Studies have indicated that hyperamnesia and partial amnesia are common for traumatic events and that the gist of the traumatic event is generally extremely well retained, while the details may be inaccurate.

✓ Hypnotic images of trauma draw from one of three sources: 1) historical events, 2) pure fantasies, or 3) a bizarre mixing of historical and fantasized elements. Apart from independent, external confirmation, there is no proven way for a therapist or client to determine the true source of a hypnotic image.

✓ There is no scientific or biblical technique that can safely and accurately unlock "repressed" events. In fact, the hypnotic techniques that are promoted are consistently shown to create highly suggestible, delusional states of mind in which clients have: 1) a decreased ability to accurately recall historical events, 2) increased experiential fantasy, and 3) increased levels of confidence in the accuracy of their recall, even though they have no reason for this.

✓ "Reasonable" hypnotic images of trauma are not necessarily any more genuine than exotic images. But they are more believable, which makes them more dangerous. The closer a delusion approximates a real scenario, has real elements and sounds "reasonable," the more difficult it is for the therapist or client to recognize it as such.

4

Stumbling Down Memory Lane

Memory, the priestess, kills the present and offers its heart to the shrine of the dead past.

SIR RABINDRANATH TAGORE, *FIREFLIES*, 1928

After taping an interview on the False Memory Crisis with *Focus on the Family* in Colorado Springs, I sat down in a side office with "Cindy" and "Tom," a young, attractive couple. Cindy heard that I was coming to do the show and requested that we get together. She began her story: "'She's very good' was the advice I got from several trusted friends. 'She has helped a lot of Christians deal with the past.'" "Dr. Lea" sounded professional; she was a licensed psychologist, and she had a graduate degree in theology. "Our first meeting went well, and Dr. Lea gave us several books to read, including *The Bondage Breaker* by Neil Anderson and *Uncovering the Mystery of MPD* by James Friesen. It all happened so fast. The next thing I knew I was in therapy several times a week. Dr. Lea hypnotized me, prayed over me, and began to demand to know who the spirits and the 'alters' were inside of me. She empowered my emotions and gave them names. Soon she didn't even call me Cindy. Instead she used the names of the alters she was finding."

Tom interrupted, "As a Christian I wasn't completely comfortable with what was happening. It seemed biblical—I mean, Dr. Lea and her helpers prayed, and they had a Bible verse for everything. Cindy was away from home more and more, though, and when she was at home she remained isolated. I was having to shoulder more of her responsibilities, and the kids were wondering what was happening to Mom. I didn't understand what was happening, and I was becoming concerned for Cindy."

Cindy continued: "I would go to see Dr. Lea, and she would hypnotize me. I don't believe in hypnosis, but she called it 'prayer visualization,' 'relaxation,' 'imagery,' so I trusted her. But they were just different names for giving over control of my will to her. Every time she prayed, it just seemed so evil. I was filled with self-hate. I would go home and cut myself with a razor blade. Every time she prayed for deliverance, I ended up with more alter personalities. I became worse, not better. I couldn't believe it when Dr. Lea told me to leave my husband and move in with another patient of hers, an MPD patient. Dr. Lea even had some Bible verse to support the idea. I asked her, 'Why? Why should I leave? Tom is a Christian, and he loves me.' Dr. Lea told me that he was interfering with my therapy."

Tom: "It's true, I was interfering. I was starting to ask questions. I have a Bible degree as well. I met with Dr. Lea, and I asked her questions that she couldn't answer from the Bible. Ultimately she told me that I would just have to trust her. That's when she started telling Cindy to leave me."

Cindy: "I was mixed up. Dr. Lea was very powerful. She could quote so many Scripture verses. She kept telling me that I was demon-possessed. I didn't feel demon-possessed. I couldn't believe I was MPD, but she was insistent that I was. I had a dear Christian friend who was questioning the memories I was reporting. She wanted to get together for lunch to talk about them. When I asked Dr. Lea if I should meet with my friend, she became enraged. 'Who is it?' she asked. 'Who is questioning me?' She took it personally. She was so furious that I didn't dare go out with my friend. Dr. Lea told me that I couldn't be friends with anyone who questioned my memories or her diagnosis of MPD."

Tom: "By then I was having some serious doubts about Dr. Lea and the whole idea of Christians having demons and alternate personalities inside of them. I could see Cindy was becoming a prisoner of therapy. She had gone to therapy to get better, but instead she was getting worse. I met with one of my pastors, against Dr. Lea's advice. The pastor didn't believe that Cindy's alters were real, and that was helpful to me. He told me to encourage Cindy to take back her life from the psychologist, to regain control of herself."

Cindy: "Therapy was getting more bizarre. Dr. Lea and her helpers would call up 'alters' and then attempt to lead them to Christ. They would pray over me for hours, sometimes in tongues. Let me tell you, the people who are into memory recovery, into MPD, into satanic ritual abuse, they really believe in what they are doing. They are persistent and dedicated to their cause."

Tom: "I do believe that Dr. Lea was well meaning. Even so, she was wrong. The therapists and pastors who are into repressed memories of abuse are hurting people and destroying families. We didn't let our church family get as close to the situation as I now know we should have. They were supportive with casseroles and flowers. They really didn't know what was happening to Cindy."

Cindy: "Yes, our church was there for us, but only so much. We have taken some time away from the church, for now. We are just stepping back and trying to figure out what is real, what is in the Bible, and what isn't."

Tom: "This has really shaken my faith to its roots. Right now all that I have left is my faith in Jesus; church programs and religion seem so shallow and so man-made. This has forced me to go deeper, to rely only upon God."

Steps for Remembering

In coming to terms with the False Memory Crisis, I started to sift through tremendous misinformation I was taught in regression seminars and readings. This included making my way back to a scientific understanding of how remembering and forgetting actually occur.

Just what is this thing we call "remembering"? There's a lot of interesting notions out there. "I've heard the brain is like a tape recorder, recording every event in a person's life." "Remembering is like rewinding a videotape. All you have to do is figure out how to rewind the brain to the right spot." "Memory is like a camera, it can capture a scene and reproduce it years later, 'picture-perfect.'" These notions about memory are quite popular. There's only one problem: they're not true.

There's a great deal of misinformation that people have about memory. That fact, in itself, is not much of a problem. I don't know much about how an automobile engine works, but I can still get in my car, turn the key, and off I go. Likewise, all of us remember and forget without having to understand how the brain manages these functions. But in issues about memory, what you don't know can hurt you. Research shows a person's beliefs about memory have a direct impact on the accuracy of their memories—for good or bad.[1]

Let me explain. If a person understands that memory is susceptible to distorting influences, they are actually better prepared to resist influences that corrupt their memories. But a person who has misbeliefs about memory (i.e., memory is "picture-perfect," isn't subject to suggestion or reconstruction) is actually left more vulnerable to the very influences they naively assume don't exist. Here's an example. Suppose you're part of an experiment in which

I'm going to hypnotize you. But before I do so, I tell you that hypnosis will make it harder for you to resist suggestions I make. Ironically, my telling you this will actually better prepare you against my influence. But what if I told you that the hypnotic technique I was going to use was a "truth enhancer" which improves your memory recall? If you believe what I've told you, research shows that you are far more likely to incorporate suggestions and fictional data into your "memories" and that your confidence in these inaccurate memories will actually increase. By telling you a lie that has put you "at ease," I've actually diminished your ability to guard against suggestions I'll be giving you.

So let's look at some of the basics of remembering and forgetting. But fair warning. This chapter is one of the more "academically challenging" you'll read in this book. But it's also one of the most important. You may have to reread a paragraph or two, but take the time to learn what's being shared. The better you're able to understand the scientific basis for how we remember and forget, the better you'll be able to defend yourself against misleading claims that are promoted in regressionism.

The first step for remembering events or information is called *encoding*. You're standing at the grocery checkout. You're putting your items on the counter, wondering where you put the checkbook, realizing two of your coupons are expired and another one is only for the twenty-four-ounce size of mouthwash, not the sixteen-ounce you have in your hand. You glance over to the magazine rack and notice headlines announcing Elvis has been discovered living in Wyoming, working at a meat-packing plant, and a live baby was found in the stomach of an alligator. In the middle of all this, your fourteen-year-old tells you that Thursday night is the church skating party and he needs a ride and ten dollars. You answer, "Uh huh," while you watch the cashier put the milk in a bag, crushing a dozen eggs that got there first. Thursday night comes and Junior strides into the living room, dressed in chic grunge fashion, announcing he's ready to go. And you say, "Go where?" With much disgust he proclaims, "I can't believe you forgot!"

Welcome to the world of "failure to encode." You see, you really didn't forget, you actually didn't remember to begin with. To remember an event, it has to get our attention, and there are plenty of things that never get there.

Most of what we remember is referred to as **explicit memory**— we are consciously aware of information that is being stored in our memory. Research also shows that we can remember information that is outside of our immediate awareness as well, something referred to as **implicit memory**. Either way, there is a short period of time that we need to transfer new information into long-term memory storage. The fact is there are tremendous volumes of information that are never registered into memory. Our ability to selectively forget some things and focus on others is actually an important survival skill. Imagine if you couldn't focus on any one thing and remembered everything from every moment of your life—what you had eaten at every meal since birth, everything that has ever been said to you, every color and texture of items in every room or shopping mall you've ever been in. This would quickly drive you into stimulus overload. The notion that the brain stores every piece of sensory awareness throughout a lifetime is an old Freudian myth—it has no basis as scientific reality.

A second aspect of remembering is that we have to occasionally **repeat** a memory in order for it to be strengthened. That's what we're doing when we study for exams, memorize people's names or learn a new phone number. When you get together with your old high school friend, both of you repeat the old stories and have a good laugh. As part of that experience you're actually refreshing your long-term memory, allowing you to recall things you've forgotten. The basic rule of thumb: the more you repeat a memory, the stronger it becomes. Without mental or verbal repetition, a memory is subject to normal processes of forgetting.

Not Quite Picture-Perfect

Ulric Neisser, a psychologist at Emory University, conducted an interesting experiment the day after the space shuttle exploded in 1986. Neisser asked 106 students to write down how, when, and where they learned about the Challenger tragedy. Three years later Neisser tracked down nearly half of the original group of students. He had them again recount how they learned about the tragedy. Neisser then compared what they wrote the first time with the account written three years later. Many of the students' memories were seriously flawed or completely wrong, yet most of them were quite certain that their three-year recall was accurate. None of the students was entirely correct, and one-third were "wildly inaccurate." Yet the "wildly inaccurate" students expressed as much certainty about the accuracy of their memories as those who were more correct.[2]

We often assume that our ability to remember is "picture-perfect." A popular view of memory is that it involves a process of "recollection," that the brain calls up a memory and "poof!" it appears perfectly intact. We just have to go to the right file and pull out a perfect recollection of an event. This simply isn't the case. Memory is actually a process of *reconstruction*, meaning the brain uses fragments of a memory that are housed in different parts of the brain and reassembles them, producing a whole "memory." What's important to understand about reconstruction is that a person's mood, mental stability, age, and beliefs, as well as events in the current environment can seriously alter how a memory is reconstructed. A specific influence is called *retrospective bias*, which occurs when we think back over past events and unknowingly change our memories with a positive "spin." We tend to focus on details that make us look particularly good and people we don't like end up looking bad. In addition, *post-event information* (things that happen later) often distort or contaminate our recollection of the original event. Elizabeth Loftus, an expert on memory research, explains:

> Truth and reality, when seen through the filter of our memories, are not objective facts but subjective, interpretive realities. We interpret the past, correcting ourselves, adding bits and pieces, deleting uncomplimentary or disturbing recollections, sweeping, dusting, tidying things up. Thus our representation of the past takes on a living, shifting reality; it is not fixed and immutable, not a place way back there that is preserved in stone, but a living thing that changes shape, expands, shrinks, and expands again, an amoebalike creature with powers to make us laugh, and cry, and clench our fists. Enormous powers—powers even to make us believe in something that never happened.[3]

Memory is also affected by *source amnesia*, a process scientists refer to when a person forgets where he saw an event (a movie, story, fantasy, or actual event) but is able to recall the scene years later. A therapist shared with me a compelling story regarding a client. One of his first memories was as a toddler. He had managed to get his head stuck under a kitchen cabinet, which was raised up off the floor on four small legs. To make matters worse, as he lay helpless his eyes adjusted to the darkness of the space and there, in the corner, he could see a coiled snake. He screamed in terror until his older sister and mother were able to free him. All his life he subsequently had a deep fear of snakes, which is certainly understandable. The only problem is, this event never happened to him. Several years ago, while this man recounted his memory with his family, his mother and sister burst out laughing. They confirmed the event was real, but it had been the older sister who experienced this trauma, not him! His confident memory was actually the product of a boy's vivid imagination. He could imagine what it was like for his sister to have her face stuck in front of a snake. Over the years, the source of the memory disappeared, but the vivid fantasy remained.

The problem is that our minds are less than perfect and each time we remember an event, we reshape it bit by bit. Because of reconstruction, retrospective bias, post-event distortion, and source amnesia our memories are inaccurate to varying degrees, even though our feelings and pride tell us otherwise.

Forgetting

"Where did I put my keys?" "What was that person's name?" "Did I turn the stove off this morning?" Everybody forgets! And we do so on a daily, moment-to-moment basis. So here's a simple question: Why do we forget things? The answer is a bit more complicated. Let's look at the standard theories on forgetting.

Decay is the oldest theory of memory loss. It's thought that memory traces in the brain gradually decay over time, like a fallen tree in a forest that is eroded by weather and natural processes. Normal metabolic processes in the body wear down a memory until it is diminished or fades completely away.

Interference theory suggests that a memory is neither lost nor damaged, an event is simply misplaced among a number of other memories that interfere with being able to recall the event later on. In this process there is *retroactive inhibition*—in which new events interrupt recall of old ones. A similar influence is *proactive inhibition*—in which the process is reversed: old events interfere with newer memories.

Cue alteration is the theory that we remember events by having "cues"—sights, sounds, and smells that allow the mind to retrieve a memory. We forget because cues are altered with the passage of time (the old neighborhood is gradually rebuilt, our childhood friends look different as we grow older).

Research reveals that forgetting involves a combination of all three theories. What research does not support is the idea that everything we've ever experienced or learned is tucked perfectly away somewhere in our brain (as Freud believed). Imagine the following scenario—you're cleaning out a box in the garage and come across one of your old algebra books. You recall that there were a series of algebra theorems you memorized back in high school. But since that time, a number of years have passed (decay), you've learned lots of other stuff (elements of interference), and you've moved to a new town and thrown away your other textbooks (cue alteration). But with this rediscovered book, you can suddenly recall a couple of the theorems that you haven't thought of for years, and you also remember what a great math student you were. The book is cuing you back to old learning and you're reviving some decaying memory traces, which includes reconstructing past events. Then you open the book and look over some of the theorems. Whoops, you got a couple of them sort of right, and two were completely off. You also pull out an old report card that shows B's and C's in math (retrospective bias). It was your friend Howard that was the math whiz, not you (source amnesia).

So here's some basic rules to remember about forgetting. Rule 1—everyone forgets. Good, bad, indifferent, we all experience memory loss. Rule 2—forgetting increases with the passage of time. The greater the interval between an event and the recalling of that event, the greater the forgetting that occurs. Rule 3—certainty can often bear little relation to accuracy. Research shows that people can be just as confident about something that is inaccurate as they are about something accurate.

It's important to keep in mind that forgetting and repression are two completely different concepts. Forgetting is a demonstrated, scientific fact that occurs according to the principles we've just discussed. Repression is a Freudian theory that maintains that the mind can instantly block out awareness of a traumatic event and recall it decades later, in complete defiance of scientific principles of remembering and forgetting.

Special Cases of Forgetting

Is it possible to forget a traumatic event? In theory, yes, but it's not very likely. Research is consistent in showing that children and adults remember emotional and traumatic events best, holding on to the *gist* of an event even if the details get fuzzy. Notice that even though Neisser's students distorted the details of the Challenger explosion, they still didn't forget that the tragedy occurred.

While normal forgetting is something we all experience, there are exotic forms that have occurred as well. These include *motivated forgetting*, *anterograde* and *retrograde amnesia*, and *fugue states*.

Motivated Forgetting

Some research suggests a person can take anxious or unacceptable thoughts and push them outside of conscious awareness. Sometimes by doing this long enough the thought is eventually lost, although it can be readily retriggered in the future. It's tempting to call this repression, but motivated forgetting involves a conscious act that takes place over a period of time and is not a foolproof method. Repression theory asserts that the blocking of a traumatic event occurs instantaneously, is involuntary, and keeps a tight seal for decades or centuries. These are important distinctions.

Anterograde and Retrograde Amnesia

Head trauma is known to create two kinds of forgetting. Anterograde involves the loss of memory for events *after* trauma to the brain. Retrograde amnesia involves loss of memory for events that occurred before an injury to the brain. Both of these types of amnesia involve physical interruptions of the brain's functions. The head trauma is an obvious event and, unlike repression, the person is acutely aware of his or her lost memories.

Fugue State

Alex is found sitting in a park in downtown Seattle. The problem is that Alex doesn't know his name, who he is, or where he's from. His amnesia is extensive and quite upsetting for him. Two days later, law enforcement is able to trace him to his family in Portland. After he arrives back home, Alex is gradually able to recover his memories of the previous eight days. What had been a financially rough year culminated into a disaster when Alex received unexpected news of his brother's death. He had been close to George and couldn't handle the shock. "Something snapped inside, and I just started walking." In a confused state, he hitchhiked his way to nowhere in particular, and finally ended up in Seattle, where authorities found him.[4]

Alex experienced a rare and controversial type of forgetting called fugue state (a type of dissociative amnesia). This is the phenomenon that is most commonly confused with Freud's notion of repression. It involves amnesia for important traumatic events which are too extensive to be explained by normal forgetting. In fugue state, it is theorized that a terrifying event is somehow able to disrupt the normal processes involved in memory encoding. This is similar to overloading the brain's circuitry, resulting in large portions of memories being disrupted and fragmented. Notice that dissociative amnesia is a very unsettling and broad experience. The person is accurately aware that he has a period of time that he can't remember, and the forgetting constitutes large portions of information, including his name, where he lives, etc.

In sharp contrast, repression theory asserts that a person can push a traumatic event out of awareness and not have the slightest notion that he has done so. A teenager could have murdered a baby, drunk its blood, danced around in black robes, and five minutes later have absolutely no recollection of anything having occurred. She then goes to bed, gets up two hours later, and aces her high-school algebra test that morning. Two nights later she does the same routine, and on it goes, countless traumatic events and she never suspects anything is wrong. Decades later, after graduating magna cum laude from Harvard, she decides to venture into regression therapy. At the coaxing of the regressionist, these traumas are "recovered" and available to be recounted perfectly. This is a radical departure from what is scientifically understood about traumatic amnesia. There simply is no evidence that this kind of highly selective, nondisruptive amnesia occurs. In fact, scientific research tells us the opposite. The more traumatic an event the more we will remember it, as in instances of posttraumatic stress disorder (which we'll discuss in a moment).

Common Questions About Memory

Now we have a basic understanding of what's involved in memory and normal and exceptional cases of forgetting. Let's get a little more specific and take a look at some commonly asked questions.

"I've read that traumatic memories are processed differently, so normal principles of memory don't apply." Sandra is a regression therapist who believes people's most traumatic memories are hidden in clusters of cells somewhere in their body. "It's almost like some part of them is locked in a time warp. Maybe it's just a set of cells

in one part of the body, but it keeps the whole body from moving forward."[5] Brent, another regressionist, explains this process. "A child's fragile psyche can be overwhelmed in moments of intense trauma, particularly those involving people they trust."[6] When this happens, the body routes the sights, smells, and sounds of the experience away from the brain and locks them in a part of the nervous system associated with the trauma. "So the person as an adult will still have a lump in their throat, and that lump actually contains the memory."[7]

Brent believes that "body memories" remain hidden for decades until the subconscious mind determines the conscious mind is ready to deal with them. At that point, the memories create pain in the area of the body where they are stored. A regressionist is able to recognize these "signals" and can then work on releasing the "memories" and alleviating the pain. This is done through the use of body massage, which frees up the memories locked in the body cells and then allows them to float back up to the brain where they can be remembered.

Another popular method is the use of natural crystals, which are rubbed on the afflicted area of the body. Regressionists believe the crystals help "unblock" the cells, allowing the memories to come forward. Brent accurately admits that there is not any scientific evidence to back up his theories. But, "For me is not to judge. . . . If a person believes enough that they have been abused, I need to work with that reality."[8]

Regressionists will often argue that the normal rules of memory that we've discussed don't apply to them or their clients. This is because they believe that traumatic events are recorded by the victims in radically different processes that overrule normal remembering and forgetting. The "trauma memory theories" go by a number of names, including "body memories," "dissociative principles," and "implicit memory systems." These different titles are simply a renaming of repression theory, which leads us back to the problem with these theories. At best, trauma models of memory are only theories—actual scientific research doesn't bear them out to be valid. To the contrary, research is consistent in showing that highly emotional events are actually more likely to be retained in memory, not less. When we know that a traumatic event has occurred, and we interview victims after the fact, we find that normal processes of memory and forgetting are occurring. Remember that theories, no matter how well worded and factual-sounding, are still theories. "Traumatic memory processing" is an artificial distinction. It's up to regression believers to prove their theoretical models, but to date they haven't done so.

"I've heard that people with post-traumatic stress disorder forget lots of things that come back to them years later in 'flashbacks.'" "Larry" is a forty-six-year-old father of two. He's single now after his second marriage fell apart three years ago. He lives alone in a small apartment and works at a job that pays the bills but little else. His drinking has been out of control for years. But it's the only thing that keeps the memories at bay. "These memories, they come and go as they please, like unwelcome guests, strolling in with blood on their feet." The ones during the night are the worst. "It always the same, I'm nineteen again, the sweat is rolling down my face, there's the bugs, and the killing." Vietnam. Back in Iowa he didn't know or care about Vietnam. But halfway around the world he finds himself living and breathing it as a young man. "Sometimes I hear the explosion, but not always. But the flash of light, the blood on my face and hands, the screaming, holding Mike's leg and trying to find the rest of him, that's always the same, that part never changes." With an exhausted look he continues, "I must have gone through this scene ten thousand times. Every time I yell out a warning to Mike, and every time, ten thousand times, the ending is the same."[9]

Highly traumatic events can sometimes lead to a condition known as post-traumatic stress disorder (PTSD). This is a condition in which a person who has experienced or witnessed a violent event will find himself reexperiencing the trauma through intrusive memories (called *flashbacks*) or dreams. Sometimes a smell, a sound, or something said will bring the trauma rushing in again, so the person will make attempts to avoid anything that might remind him of, or "cue," a memory. He usually experiences trouble sleeping, irritability, difficulty concentrating, and *hypervigilance* (being constantly alert to any potential danger). Notice that a person suffering from PTSD doesn't forget his trauma. Dr. Paul Ingmundson is a psychologist at a Texas Veterans Hospital. For fifteen years he has worked as a specialist with war veterans who are recovering from post-traumatic stress disorder. "In all my years of working with PTSD, the thing I've noticed is that my patients have always remembered their war traumas. It's never been like what the regressionists talk about, where somebody suddenly remembers something twenty years later. Really, it's the opposite. These guys just can't forget what happened, though they wish they could."[10]

Many regressionists argue that their clients are experiencing PTSD symptoms and then use hypnotic techniques to do "archeological digging." For example, a regressionist points to various symptoms in a client's life as indications of PTSD that are related to space alien abduction, even though the client doesn't remember any space aliens. Then, in hypnosis, the client develops hypnotic fantasies of space aliens that confirm the original diagnosis of PTSD. This is a dangerous form of circular reasoning, one that I regularly applied with my clients concerning sexual abuse.

Now stop for a moment and think. This brings up an important point of logic and sequencing. Event "A" may lead to result "X." But it doesn't necessarily work the other way around. There's a person who is skiing and accidentally breaks his leg ("A" leads to "X"). But not every broken leg is because of a skiing accident ("X" can be caused by lots of possibilities). A person's sexual abuse can lead to symptoms of PTSD, but symptoms of PTSD are not always because of sexual abuse. Symptoms mistaken to be PTSD can actually be caused by certain mental and personality disorders (we'll discuss these in Chapter 10). In science we refer to this as a failure to provide an appropriate *differential diagnosis:* Symptoms can point to a number of possible disorders that have to be ruled out. So here's the rule to remember: The diagnosis of PTSD requires a freestanding memory of a traumatic event, not the other way around.

"What about people who have retrieved memories from infancy or their mothers' wombs?" "Gale" is a thirty-eight-year-old Christian who believes she is the victim of sexual and satanic abuse by her father and mother. In our conversations she revealed how regression therapy helped her to recall the brutal assaults Dad and Mom had inflicted on her in infancy. In fact, she was even able to go back into her mother's womb and remember hateful words her parents spoke about her. Ultimately, she was able to travel back in time to before she was born, where she had conversations with "God" and could clearly see "God" holding her and preparing her to be born into this life. Gale expressed confidence in her fantasies because she had prayed to the "Holy Spirit" and believed He revealed these to her—"He never would have misled me." Based on her fantasies, Gale has completely cut off any contact with her family. Living alone, left without any family, Gale has only the support and friendship of others in her regression group.

Interestingly, 54 percent of therapists believe that they can retrieve memories from infancy[11] and a recent national survey has revealed shocking results—68 percent of repressed memory claims are said to have occurred prior to the age of four.[12] Are Gale and other regression believers right? Are there thousands of infant and childhood memories somewhere within you, perfectly preserved in suspended animation? Can we go back even further, to the fallopian tube, prior to being conceived?

The notion that we can recover memories from infancy or the womb is exotic and holds great appeal for many. But the fact of the matter is there is simply no scientific basis for these inviting beliefs. We need physical brain maturity in order to transfer information from short-term memory storage over to long-term memory. Just as the development of the human body requires about one-and-a-half decades to complete, so also the human brain continues its development for a few years after birth. The hypocampus, which is involved in the transfer of short-term memory to long-term storage, is still developing in infancy. Myelination is a protective sheath that covers the brain cell axons. Without it, a large portion of the electrical impulses that are transferred between brain cells are lost. The myelination process is not complete for the first year of life. Bottom line, studies of childhood memory consistently show that people's earliest, reliable memories do not date back before the age of about four.[13]

These aspects of brain development may sound academic, but the implications are practical. Gale believes that she has recovered memories of trauma from her infancy, including digital rape by her mother. But these "memories" introduce several problems. As an infant Gale would have to distinguish between someone changing her diaper, taking her temperature rectally, cleaning and washing her, a difficult bowel movement, and digital rape. After such advanced sensory awareness, she would then need to transfer this short-term memory into long-term storage. But she won't have a developed hypocampus, completed myelination process, or language to encode the event for the next couple of years. Next, she would need to go for several decades without rehearsing the memory and then bring it up pristine and perfect at the prompting of her regressionist, in defiance of all that we know about forgetting. Her fantasies of being with God before her conception have no basis in reality, but Gale's claims of abuse and previous life were accepted as truth by well-meaning therapists and Christians in her hometown.

"What about people who can't remember periods of time during their childhoods? Isn't that a sign that something is wrong?" There is a lot

of talk about *memory gaps*. A common misconception I was taught was the idea that memory gaps in a person's childhood indicate that something was wrong during that missing time period. This is one of the more popular "indicators" that there are repressed memories lurking in a person's unconscious, one that I regularly used to convince clients something was hidden inside them. In my zeal I had ignored my training as a psychologist. You see, in psychology we call these "gaps" the *infantile amnesiac barrier*. It is very common and normal for people to have memory gaps from their childhood, even up to age ten or twelve. These gaps are due to physical and developmental issues that impede memory retention and lead to memory loss, which we discussed earlier. Dr. John Kihlstrom, a cognitive psychologist and professor at Yale University, explains, "Our memories of our childhood are impoverished, not by trauma, but by the simple facts of cognitive development. Kids just don't have the equipment to remember."[14] Common sense also gives us some clues. For each of us, the events of our childhood represent our oldest memories. In comparison to last summer's vacation, what you did in first grade is subject to much more memory loss. It only makes sense that our oldest memories are the least complete and most inaccurate.

"You just can't make up a traumatic event." Many of the regressionists I've talked to argue that it's one thing to admit that memory loss and retrospective bias can distort details of a traumatic event, but it's quite another matter to argue that an entirely fictional event can be created in a client's mind. "I mean, a client recovers the memory of her rape that occurred thirty years ago. Maybe she gets the colors of the curtains wrong, but she certainly can't make the whole thing up. The core of the memory is what's important, not the details," one might suggest.

That's a good point and certainly what I believed when I was promoting regression therapy. But following this line of reasoning, we must assume that all, each and every one, of the recovered memories of space alien abductions, past lives, womb traumas, sexual abuses, and ritual tortures are real because "the mind can't make up such things." This much we know for certain: Of the thousands of cases of recovered "memories," we can safely conclude that a large portion of hypnotic fantasies do not have a basis in reality, something that even the most hard-core promoter of regression will reluctantly admit.

The fact is, everyone's mind is very capable of creating detailed and very emotional events that are absolutely fictional. It's called dreaming. Remember that nightmare you had several years ago? It was so vivid and terrifying. You woke with a start and found yourself staring into the darkness, sweating, breathing heavily. For a moment it seemed so real, but now, thankfully, you're awake and the dream is passing. Or how about during the day when you find yourself sitting at your desk, bored. Your mind turns to adventure, exotic places, being a rock musician, whatever. For a few minutes you get to drift away to some other time and place and have some fun. Then it's back to mundane reality at hand.

Our imagination is a powerful gift. With it we can dream beautiful dreams and imagine wonderful possibilities. But this same gift can be turned toward negative purposes, imagining dark and fearful events, dwelling on hurts. Our imagination is able to create vivid, detailed scenes that produce within us joy, anger, tears, or sexual arousal. You name it, we can imagine it. Our thoughts have very real consequences in our lives. One of the things that happens when imagination goes awry is called a *delusion*. People can come to believe hurtful, terrifying fantasies are real and in the process harm themselves and others. In one study, a researcher implanted the idea of reincarnation in numerous subjects. He scripted out several "past-life" scenarios and then made subtle suggestions to subjects while they were under hypnosis. They were able to experience these scripts as real and produce intricate details of their "past lives."[15] Elizabeth Loftus, one of the world's leading experts on memory, successfully implanted the idea in subjects that they had been lost in a shopping mall as a child. She first checked with the subjects' families to be sure the subjects hadn't really had this experience in childhood. She then enlisted family members' help. They were to confirm the implanted idea if the subject asked them about it. Then Loftus, without the aid of hypnosis, suggested that the subjects had been lost in the mall as children. At first the subjects were uncertain. But as might be expected, after a brief passage of time the subjects not only accepted the implanted idea as real, but even added fine detail and emotional effect when later describing the experience.[16]

Then there's the case of the Ingram family. Paul Ingram was arrested for satanic ritual abuse in 1988, based upon the recovered fantasies of his two daughters. They had been prayed over by a Christian "prophet" who had diagnosed them as having been abused even though they had no memory of having been so. Erika accused first, her sister later, at her prompting. Initially Ingram remembered nothing, but he was convinced that his daughters, both strong Christians, could never lie. Later, after intense police interrogation, and the "counsel" of his pastor/counselor (who told him he was demonized) Paul began to enter into trance-states of mind and produced fantasies of how he had ritually and sexually abused his children. He sincerely believed (coached by the pastor and police) that if he confessed and pled guilty, then he would be released from the demonic power, be able to recall the crimes himself, and his daughters would feel safe and begin their own recovery.

In the midst of these proceedings Richard Ofshe, a University of California (Berkeley) sociologist, was brought in by the *prosecution* to further the case against Ingram. From the outset, Ofshe had his doubts about the veracity of these recovered fantasies. Ofshe decided to test Ingram's suggestibility, since suggestion and accusation over long periods of interrogation was the primary factor in eliciting a confession from him. Ofshe made up a story about Ingram forcing two of his children to have sex together. Ofshe checked with the children involved, to be sure that the event never happened. Ofshe then confronted Ingram with the fictional story and asked him to write a description of how it happened. Ingram returned to his cell, prayed and hours later produced a detailed written account of the events Ofshe implanted. When Ofshe confronted Ingram with the truth, Ingram did not believe him, insisting that Ofshe was wrong and the event really occurred!

It was too late for Ingram. Though the stories didn't match those of his daughters very closely and there was no corroborating evidence, he pled guilty and, without a trial, was sentenced to twenty years to life. It was only after he was transferred to the state prison, where he was away from the toxic influence of his interrogators and his pastor/counselor, that Ingram began to think critically and realized he had made it all up. But there is hope, a national effort is under way to have Paul Ingram tried in a court of law, a basic human right that he was denied.[17]

On a lighter note, Peter J. Reveen, a stage hypnotist, recounts several events that have occurred while performing his hypnotism show:

> In suggesting to a stage full of volunteers that they are going to relive "past lives," I carefully avoid giving the impression that I have any doubts about the reality of reincarnation, for then a sizable number of volunteers would pick up on my disbelief,

and fail to fantasize at all. . . . Consequently, night after night, dozens of volunteers give detailed, entertaining descriptions of imagined past lives, that are partly dormant memories from their present lives, partly elaborations of historical books and movies . . . and pure fantasy. . . . In one show two men at the same time claimed to be King Henry VIII of England. Clearly, for either one to be recalling a genuine former incarnation, the other must have been fantasizing. Another time two subjects, a man and a woman, both claimed to be Christopher Columbus. And once, in 1985, I even had a subject "regress" to a past life in which he was Prince Charles, husband of Diana and son of Queen Elizabeth II [who is still alive].[18]

Let's be clear about this point. Everyone is capable of creating fantasies that look and feel real. Some are just better at it than others, and these are called Fantasy-Prone personalities and patients with Grade Five Syndrome, which we'll discuss in Chapter 10.

"There are lots of recovered memories that people get without the help of a therapist. Aren't these more valid?" This is one of the more common arguments that I hear from regression believers. Interestingly, the majority of space alien abductees have remembered their abductions away from therapy. So the question is, doesn't that make them valid? Researchers have noted that space alien abductees have something in common—an active belief in space aliens *prior* to recovering memories of space aliens.[19] It is only subsequent to this belief that they are able to experience their fantasies of abduction and experimentation by space aliens. This was consistent with my experience as well—typically, "spontaneous memory recovery" occurred only after a client had been exposed to regression teachings and started to believe in them. In Chapter 8 we'll discuss the importance of a preexisting belief system ("I'll see it when I believe it"), media influences, and how someone can experience vivid fantasies in the form of hypnagogic and hypnopompic hallucinations. Another key point to understand is that people are capable of hypnotizing themselves, referred to as creating a *self-induced trance*. The bottom line is that fantasies experienced in self-induced trance are no more valid than those guided by therapists.

Points to Remember

✓ Memory is a process of *reconstruction*, not recollection. *Retrospective bias, post-event information,* and *source amnesia* can distort our reconstruction of a historical event.

✓ There are several basic steps to recording an event in memory. First, we need physical brain maturity; second, we have to encode an event; and finally, we have to occasionally repeat a memory in order for it to be strengthened.

✓ In memory research there are some basic rules to keep in mind. Rule 1: Everyone forgets things. Rule 2: Forgetting increases with the passage of time. Rule 3: Certitude is not always related to accuracy. Rule 4: We tend to remember emotional and traumatic events best, holding on to the gist of an emotional event, while the details become distorted. Theories for normal forgetting include *memory decay, cue alteration,* and *source amnesia*. Less common sources include *motivated forgetting, anterograde* and *retrograde amnesia,* and *fugue state* (which is often confused with repression).

✓ Highly traumatic events can sometimes lead to a condition known as post-traumatic stress disorder (PTSD) in which a person is recurrently plagued with memories of his or her trauma (without a period of forgetting). In diagnosing PTSD, it is essential that there is a freestanding memory of trauma.

✓ It is normal for people to have memory gaps (called the *infantile amnesiac barrier*) in their childhoods, even up to age ten or twelve. Memory gaps are *not* necessarily an indication that anything traumatic has occurred in one's childhood.

✓ Everyone's mind is capable of creating detailed and emotional events that are fictional. Healthy examples include dreaming and fantasy, while pathological instances include paranoid delusions and hypnotic hypersuggestibility.

✓ Hypnotic images that are experienced apart from therapy due to self-induced trance are no more reliable than those "discovered" in therapist-induced trance.

Satanic Panic

There are two equal and opposite errors into which our race can fall about the devils. One is to disbelieve in their existence. The other is to believe, and to feel an excessive and unhealthy interest in them. They themselves are equally pleased by both errors, and hail a materialist or a magician with the same delight.

C. S. LEWIS, *THE SCREWTAPE LETTERS*, 1941

They were the experts. They—they were the experts. They said, 'We've been studying this for fifteen years. We've done the research.'" "Wendy" went into a psychiatric hospital with anxiety attacks. In her first session with a regression therapist she was diagnosed as a "polyfragmented multiple." It was explained that she was like a vase that had been dropped on a cement floor, shattering into thousands of pieces. Who she thought she was, was a lie. Her real self contained dozens of different personalities, splinters of the original "vase." Her regressionist was nationally known for his pioneering work with multiple personality disorder (MPD) and it was his job to glue her back together. What Wendy never suspected was that his glue job would take her into an unspeakable hell of years of "therapy" that would cost two-and-a-half million dollars and rob her of her family.

How had Wendy ended up in this pottery shop? She had a difficult background, health problems, and a recovering alcoholic husband. Life was tough, but Wendy was dealing with these problems. A good friend described her as having a healthy relationship with her husband and son, and that she was a great mom with lots of patience. Yet she kept on having these panic attacks and sometimes the fears and doubts seemed overwhelming. Could it be that there were deeper underlying issues? She attended a nine-week series on Cults in America at a large church. Here she heard the pastor's admonition that, *"Satan worshipers pose the greatest threat to our society,"* which started her musing on potential root causes to her depression and anxiety.

After therapy began the gluing process got progressively stickier. It seemed that the doctors knew more about Wendy's family than she did. She was identified as a fifth-generation cult member and was cult royalty. She was heavily medicated with a myriad of drugs and was frequently hypnotized. Wendy's world began to crack. Everything was black, everything was fear. She was told that she had been programmed to self-destruct if she revealed cult secrets, that she was the only one in five generations who was given the insight to break the cycle, and that she must continue treatment for the sake of her son. She was told that she had killed people and abused children horribly. She was supposed to be part of an international network of evil satanists, as well as being a spy from the cult. Eventually the regressionists convinced her that she was planning to kill her husband and son.

"David," her son, was also admitted to the hospital, diagnosed as a "structured, polyfragmented MPD" who had been programmed for suicide, homicide, and returning to the cult. A nurse who cared for him on the children's ward described him as *a normal little boy who was full of joy, full of activity, very normal, talented little kid.* He was ten years old.

Wendy described her life "*. . . as a snake pit. As hell. I was sure I was going to die there. And yet, I had doubts all the way. My journal is just full of statements like, 'This can't be true. I've just made all this up.'*" Finally, her insurance company started pushing for a change of status, and Wendy took this moment to refuse treatment. "*I decided that I had nothing to lose. I decided I just wanted to leave and take my chances.*" Wendy had no more money. She was released on the condition that she find a sophisticated security system to protect herself from the cult, and that she find a competent therapist.

Miraculously she found one. On the second visit, he asked her, "*Do you like being a multiple personality?*" She answered, "*No, I hate it. You know I'm working really hard to integrate all of these parts.*" His simple response was amazing. "*You don't have to be a multiple anymore. You can just stop. Just stop. Stop working. Stop thinking about it. We'll just get you physically healthy and off this medication.*" And just like that, the insanity stopped. Wendy sums it up. "*I went through withdrawal. I was in awful physical shape. But when I stopped working on the memories, they—it just dissipated. The memories stopped. No one shot at me. I could make phone calls. I never got poisoned. Nothing happened.*"

Wendy made her way out of the torture, but her family didn't. Her husband and son still believe the "experts," who are now millions of dollars richer for their little glue job, which destroyed this family. Wendy is left with an emptiness, a void that nothing can fill. In subsequent legal action, the court stated it "*firmly believes that Wendy's initial difficulties were not a manifestation of multiple disorders secondary to ritualistic abuse.*" The hospital settled the lawsuit for a massive amount of money, but that is small consolation for the years of torture she endured and the ongoing loss of her family.[1]

Old Habits Die Hard

Wendy represents only one case of thousands of patients who have been convinced that they were raised in multigenerational satanic cults. Here's another Satanic Ritual Abuse (SRA) story you might have read about.

In '92 one of the most sensational cases of satanic ritualistic abuse in the United States was discovered. Seventeen girls from a small East Coast community exhibited traumatic symptoms consistent with post-traumatic stress disorder. Experts were called in to examine the girls. While initially unable to recall what had occurred, the girls were eventually able to recover repressed memories of ritual abuse. Before the investigation was over, the largest SRA scandal to date had been uncovered, and 140 people were indicted in the subsequent investigation. Though there was no actual evidence of SRA, the authorities found the testimony of the girls to be compelling and convincing. Local community leaders were stunned that this could occur in their town without anyone suspecting.

Of the 140 people that were originally indicted, thirty-one were found guilty of ritualistic abuse. Of those found guilty, eleven were sentenced to prison and served varying amounts of prison time, nineteen of the guilty were hanged, and one man was slowly crushed between huge stones until his death two days later.

The year, of course, was *1692*. The place was Salem, Massachusetts.

Between 1484 and 1723 approximately two hundred thousand people were tortured and murdered during waves of witch hysteria, which cycled across various European countries. Typically a community would become panicked that there were witches causing various calamities (hailstorms, cows giving sour milk, young girls with unexplained afflictions, etc.). Ministers preached against the horrors of the witches and the need for God's people to ferret out evildoers and bring them to confession and justice. Magical lists of "indicators" were developed that allowed God's faithful to detect a witch. After torture with some of the cruelest techniques ever devised, the accused would admit guilt or die during the proceedings. The confessions were then used as proof that the original "indicators" were correct. Shortly after confessing, the accused was murdered (typically strangled, hanged, or beheaded) and burned. The witch panic would progress, leaving in its wake up to thousands murdered in a particular region before it would eventually subside. Often the satanic panic would resurface decades later in the same community and the cycle would start anew.

Three hundred years later, the witch-hunters are back in full force, looking for new victims. *Webster's Third International Dictionary* defines a witch-hunt as, "An investigation of or campaign against dissenters conducted on the pretext of protecting the public welfare and resulting in public persecution and defamation of character."[2]

In a definitive work on witch hysterias of the past, Rossell Robbins noted aspects of inquisitional laws that were created to guarantee that the accused would be found guilty.[3] His historical review was published in 1960, yet perfectly describes today's False Memory Crisis:

Convictions in the Witch Trials	Today's Convictions in Regressionists' Offices
1. The procedure was secret.	1. The development and confirmation of abusive fantasies are done under the guise of "client confidentiality" and the parents are never allowed a defense.
2. Rumors were accepted as an indication of guilt, which the accused had to disprove.	2. Unsubstantiated fantasies of abuse are accepted as indicators of guilt, which parents have the burden of disproving.
3. Frequently the precise charges were concealed from the accused.	3. The large majority of parents don't know the specific crimes they are accused of committing. Their accusing child assumes the parent already knows, and the therapist maintains confidentiality.

4. Persons normally debarred from giving evidence in all other trials were permitted and encouraged to testify in witch trials—children of ten years and younger, perjurers, felons, and excommunicates.
5. No favorable evidence was permitted about the accused's previous life and character.
6. A witness for the accused would be presumed to be a friend, and therefore guilty by association of the same crime.
7. The most severe torture was reserved to make the accused an informer; often the names of "accomplices" were suggested to him by the judges or hangmen.
8. No one accused was ever found innocent. At best, his case would be declared Not Proven, and the trial could be reopened at any time. However, this was theoretical, for in practice the accused was tortured until he confessed or died.

4. Severely mentally disturbed patients are always assumed to be describing real events in their fantasies, including those they describe when regressed into infancy or the womb.
5. Any evidence of the parents' integrity or Christian character is reinterpreted as a perpetrator's clever disguise.
6. Anyone who defends the accused is also "in denial" and accused of being an accomplice as well.
7. With a macabre twist, the therapist is able to suggest potential abusers to the hypnotized patient, who then incorporates the suggestions into her fantasies.
8. Once accused, the parents are never able to clear their names. Therapists, accusing children, lifelong friends, and church members assume that the needed evidence has simply disappeared decades ago in an attempted cover-up.

When I was practicing regressionism, I deeply believed in multigenerational satanists. Through different seminars and readings, I had learned deep, intricate conspiracy theories about them. With their legions of followers, immense wealth, and tremendous power, they were the "unseen hand" that guides the events of nations. The notion appealed to my beliefs as a Christian in an actual Satan. It seemed to explain so much of what was wrong with our world. I listened to national "experts" teach with hushed tones about intricate theories and expound on horrific crimes satanists were committing.

The more popular version teaches that multigenerational satanists are believed to have existed for centuries and thousands of them have infiltrated positions of power throughout the world. In their worship and service to Satan, they torture and murder thousands of adults and children each year. They also have ancient, magical techniques that they use in their rituals to create *alter personalities* in helpless victims. In regression circles these "victims" are identified as suffering from multiple personality disorder. It's interesting to note that before therapy the client has no knowledge of the other personalities within her. Regressionists believe the knowledge of the cult is locked away in one or more of the hidden personalities, and the regressionist is the only one who can uncover the secret past by the use of different hypnotic techniques. Like the earlier witch hunts, the conspiracy theories have an anti-Semitic theme, maintaining that Jewish mystics (who are allegedly multigenerational satanists) were smuggled out of Nazi Germany by the CIA and then taught undercover law enforcement how to create alter personalities in helpless victims. Since then the CIA has also supposedly used these techniques.

The multigenerational satanists are said to be so advanced that they are able to plant "triggers" in the victim, so that decades later the victim can be preprogrammed to kill herself on a particular anniversary or return to the cult if she ever discovers the truth of her past. So, once in therapy, the regressionist will forbid the client from reading any mail or accepting any calls from family members because at any moment a trigger word can be read or heard and the client will then kill herself or drop out of therapy and return to the cult. Regressionists estimate anywhere from 200,000 up to 500,000 people have survived the multigenerational satanists' tortures and secretly carry the knowledge of the cult and the implanted triggers outside of conscious awareness.

With all this talk there must be something to the conspiracy theories.

Or is there?

Types of Satanists

In today's society, there are generally four types of satanists identified. The first are described as *dabblers* or *dressers*. These are the adolescents and adults who take on the garb, speech, and appearance of satanism because they like the sense of power, group affiliation, and "startle effect" it provides. The second group is the *self-styled satanists* who are more active and dangerous. They do indeed kill animals and sometimes humans. But they are independent, small groups or individuals that lack ties to any major movement or network. Rather than actual satanists, typically this group of people practices variations of Senteria, a mixture of voodoo and Christian rituals popular in South America. A third group is the *religious satanists*. These are the people who practice the satanic faith, i.e., the Church of Satan in San Francisco, which was founded by Anton LeVay. The key point in understanding these first three groups is that they are recognized, active, and evidence for their existence is well established. It is the fourth group, *multigenerational satanists*, that represents the controversy for the Christian community and law enforcement.

I was recently a guest on *Focus on the Family* with Dr. James Dobson. As we discussed different aspects of the False Memory Crisis, another guest on the show, a psychiatrist, remarked that satanic ritual abuse is a serious, widespread problem in the United States. In fact, his chain of psychiatric clinics had even opened up a special treatment facility in Chicago to help victims of SRA. He noted that just the week before he had a client who had recovered memories of delivering a baby and sacrificing it at a satanic cult. He insisted that her story was true, even verifiable.

Dr. Dobson's reply to this guest was intriguing: A few years before Dobson had served on the attorney general's Board on Missing and Exploited Children. The Board sought to determine just how widespread satanic cult activity was and how prevalent were incidents of children being sacrificed. Dobson noted that of all the cases that they had investigated, there was only one which the FBI had verified as a ritual sacrifice.

So who's right? Are there, as the sincere psychiatrist contends, thousands of victims of multigenerational satanic cults, so many in fact that they warrant a special treatment center? Or is Dr. Dobson correct, that ritual abuses are exceedingly rare?

Randy Emon is a recently retired police sergeant who served twenty years on the force in southern California. He spent a number of years as the president of C.O.I.N. (Christian Occult Investigator's Network), has trained police officers across the nation in how to investigate occult-related crime, and has appeared in a number of documentaries on SRA. He describes his story:[4]

In 1985 I began to investigate occult-related crimes. For the next six and a half years I collected evidence. I found hard evidence to verify the existence of dabblers, religious satanists, and self-styled satanists. However, a fourth group was spoken of over and over, and it was the most fascinating: multigenerational satanists. Though I didn't find any hard facts or even corroborative evidence for the existence of this group, I allowed myself to believe that they were too smart to leave any evidence behind.

Generational satanists are the group identified by "ritual abuse survivors" as their tormentors and abusers. As an investigator, I devoted most of my time to investigating this fourth group of satanists. I attended seminars, where I listened to survivors relay stories of abuse at the hands of grandparents, parents, schoolteachers, neighbors, and even policemen, all as members of secret, multigenerational satanic cults. I interviewed hundreds of people who reported that they had "bred" to supply babies for sacrifice by the cults they were raised in, that they had been married to the devil in hideous ceremonies, and that they were still being followed and tormented by satanists. Sad to say, I began to believe that multigenerational satanists existed and that they were supernaturally able to keep themselves hidden. I bought into the hysteria completely. Even so, down inside, something still bothered me.

Between 1988 and 1991 the media paid a lot of attention to the stories of SRA. I had interviewed many of these "survivors" and began to notice a striking similarity between the stories I was hearing.

- Each person had emotional problems for which he or she sought counseling.
- After lengthy counseling, many were eventually diagnosed as ritual abuse survivors, often with MPD.
- In almost all cases the use of hypnosis or regression was reported in order to get to the "memories" of satanic abuse.
- None was able to offer any proof to verify his or her story.
- Upon investigation their stories were not corroborated, and were often conclusively proven to be impossible and untrue.
- Belief in their stories was used as criteria for selection of friends and associates. Nonbelief or skepticism (even asking

for objective proof) was seen as "not believing" and almost always resulted in rejection of the disbeliever (often with the encouragement and support of their therapist and other survivors).

By 1992 I had trained over five thousand police officers to be aware of occult elements in crimes that they were investigating. But a doubt was growing inside of me and I made an important decision: I decided to discontinue teaching my police courses until I resolved my growing doubts.

I inquired in a number of places in order to find answers. I found some interesting facts. One of the first things I came across were accounts of space alien abduction. What fascinated me was the striking similarity to ritual abuse survivor stories.

- Initially, both developed bad dreams, usually paranoid in nature.
- Neither group of survivors remembered specific details of their past until they sought counseling for an existing emotional problem.
- The therapist always utilized hypnosis or visualization techniques. When groups were involved their memories were quite similar.
- Females in each group claim to have been seduced, often for breeding purposes. Many claimed their children were subsequently killed or kidnapped.
- Both groups describe special rooms where they had to disrobe, were fastened to a table, and then subjected to ritual cutting, sexual violation, examination, or surgery.
- Both groups struggle with believing their recalled events, often relying upon other survivors or therapists for emotional support and validation.

I was in contact with many police organizations in the western United States. I knew most of the police investigators who specialized in occult crime investigation. As I talked to them I found out that a lot of them were having the same doubts I was. Many had rejected the idea of satanic abuse as unprovable and probably pure fantasy. Some had never believed, due to the lack of any evidence. Some, like Ken Lanning at the FBI, were subject to intense criticism for telling the truth. So there it was. None of us found any evidence of multigenerational satanism.

I had been featured in eight documentaries on satanism. I had conducted dozens of television interviews and appearances. I had testified in court as an occult expert. Then I reversed my opinion. The phone stopped ringing. No one wanted interviews anymore. I didn't have any more horror stories to repeat. Survivors were sure that satanists had gotten to me, but it was the truth that had opened my eyes. When I let blind belief overrule objectivity, I missed the mark. Like the young man who noticed the king lacked any clothing, I decided to report the truth, even though it was not easy.

People who believe that there is a secret conspiracy of multigenerational satanists need to investigate what they are believing and reporting to others. They need to seek the truth. I did, and it led me back to truth and the ability to objectively question these stories.

Randy Emon mentions Kenneth Lanning, a supervisory special agent with the Federal Bureau of Investigation at the National Center for the Analysis of Violent Crime. He specializes in investigating cases of violent acts toward children. After eighteen years of researching, training, and consulting, he concludes that there is little or no corroborative evidence of massive SRA abuse networks:

Until hard evidence is obtained and corroborated, the public should not be frightened into believing that babies are being bred and eaten, that 50,000 missing children are being murdered in human sacrifices, or that satanists are taking over America's day care centers or institutions. No one can prove with absolute certainty that such activity has *not* occurred. The burden of proof, however, as it would be in a criminal prosecution, is on those who claim that it has occurred. The explanation that the satanists are too organized and law enforcement is too incompetent only goes so far in explaining the lack of evidence. For at least eight years American law enforcement has been aggressively investigating the allegations of victims of ritual abuse. There is little or no evidence for the portion of their allegations that deals with large-scale baby breeding, human sacrifice, and

organized satanic conspiracies. Now it is up to mental health professionals, not law enforcement, to explain why victims are alleging things that don't seem to have happened.[5]

Save the Children

Men become superstitious, not because they have too much imagination, but because they are not aware that they have any.

GEORGE SANTAYANA, *LITTLE ESSAYS*, 1920

Dramatic claims are often used to promote beliefs about multigenerational satanism and child abductions. For example, Representative Paul Simon told a House committee that a "conservative estimate . . . [is that] 50,000 children [are] abducted by strangers annually."[6] Child Find, a child search organization, estimated that only 10 percent of these children are recovered, another 10 percent are found dead, and the remaining forty thousand per year remain missing.[7] Dr. Al Carlisle says forty thousand to sixty thousand people are killed in satanic rituals each year.[8] SRA "survivors" and lecturing regressionists rely on these kinds of statements to prove that children are missing in large numbers and that many of these children end up on satanic altars.

But everything isn't quite as regressionists have made it out to be. Bob and Gretchen Passantino are an investigative team in California who run Answers In Action, a Christian ministry that focuses on exposing the occult and educating Christians about fraudulent claims. On the topic of tens of thousands of missing children, they note:

When statistical studies on missing children are examined, we find that the truth does not fit the SRA conspiracy model. In fact, the vast majority of children reported missing each year are accounted for within a twelve-month period, leaving fewer than 300 unaccounted for after one year. The majority of missing children either are taken by noncustodial parents in custody disputes or are runaways. Certainly to a parent whose child is missing, the size of the problem is immaterial, the grief real, and the suffering profound. But it is wrong to confuse compassion for a blind acceptance of false statistics in a futile effort to bolster an SRA conspiracy theory.[9]

The U.S. Department of Justice, in a definitive review of this subject, has shown that on average 52 to 158 children are murdered by strangers each year in the United States.[10] Where are the thousands of children that are supposed to be missing? Truth is, they aren't. But the regressionists have done such an effective job of instilling satanic panic that many of us within the church have come to firmly believe that thousands of helpless victims are missing and have been murdered. The Passantinos note:

> Since 1989, we have done a thorough investigation of Satanic Ritual Abuse (SRA), interviewed hundreds of people who believe they are adult survivors and interviewed almost all of the principals on both sides of the issue. . . . We are convinced that the bulk of the SRA phenomenon is the result of directed, inappropriate therapeutic technique and not a reflection of what is actually happening in the real world.[11]

Are the Passantinos just wishful thinkers? Have they been fooled? The most comprehensive study on evidence for multigenerational satanism was completed in 1994 by the National Center on Child Abuse and Neglect. Researchers conducted a survey of over eleven thousand psychiatrists, psychologists, clinical social workers, district attorneys, police departments, and social-service agencies and accumulated over twelve thousand reported accusations of ritual abuse that had been investigated. The researchers noted: "Since the McMartin preschool case, there have been claims of ritualistic and sadistic child abuse in cases all over the country, and we've been concerned. The survey was to see just how well-founded these concerns are—if these are just based on mistaken perceptions or there is some firm evidence."[12] The researchers also noted, "Over the last decade, accusations of molesting by cults have been made in thousands of cases and in retrospective claims by adult patients in psychotherapy who say they were abused as children. Combined with sensationalistic press coverage, these lawsuits and other reports have led many people to believe that there is a nationwide network of satanic groups preying on the young."[13]

The survey found occasional cases of lone abusers who used ritualistic trappings. There was "convincing evidence of lone perpetrators or couples who say they are involved with Satan or use the claim to intimidate victims."[14] But in the thousands of cases investigated, not a single case related to well-organized satanic rings was shown to be true. "After scouring the country, we found no evidence for large-scale cults that sexually abuse children."[15] The survey showed that "there was not a single case where there was clear corroborating evidence for the most common accusation, that there was a well-organized, intergenerational Satanic cult, who sexually molested and tortured children in their homes or schools for years and committed a series of murders."[16]

The researchers continued:

> There are, of course, people who will be unswayed by this new study because of their belief that abusive satanic groups do exist but are successful at eluding detection. But previous smaller studies done by the Michigan State Police, the Virginia Crime Commission, the Office of the Attorney General in Utah and the British Government had similar findings. Many psychotherapists who have been vocal about a supposed epidemic of sexual abuse by well-organized satanic rings have grown more cautious of late.[17]

Dr. Bennett Braun, a psychiatrist, summarized, "There's clearly been a contagion, a contamination of what people say in therapy because of what they see on TV or read about satanic ritual abuse."[18]

Rumors

Rumor goes forth at once, Rumor than whom
No other speedier evil thing exists;
She thrives by rapid movement, and acquires
Strength as she goes; small at the first from fear,
She presently uplifts herself aloft,
And stalks upon the ground and hides her head
Among the clouds.
VIRGIL, *AENEID*, 30-19 B.C.

During the early 1980s a popular rumor circulated in America that maintained that Proctor & Gamble, producer of a large assortment of household items, was run by satanists. Versions of the story had the company president on a popular TV talk show in which he revealed that Proctor & Gamble tithed 10 percent of their profits to the Church of Satan. The rumors spread like wildfire. Occult "experts" said they were able to decipher 666, the Mark of the Beast, in the corporation's emblem. Churches began to organize boycotts, and the company received thousands of phone calls a month wanting to know if they really were Satan's servants. During this same time I was a student at a small, conservative Bible college in California. I watched fellow students come together to discuss the latest news they had heard. Prayer groups were organized to counteract Satan's bold advances. We were scared, angered, and excited. There was only one problem.

The stories weren't true.

No Proctor & Gamble president had appeared on a talk show, the corporation emblem was over a century old and had no references to Satan. Nobody was tithing money to the Church of Satan. They had done no wrong, but Proctor & Gamble had to spend immense amounts of money to calm the rumors. Where had these rumors come from? Subsequent investigations revealed that the rumors originated in the conservative Bible Belt of the southern United States, where pastors had taught the rumors from their pulpits.[19] The rumors continue to circulate. Like the witch-hunters from three hundred years ago, zealous Christians have used the pulpit to spread satanic panic.

Have you heard about the "vanishing hitchhiker," in which a stranger is picked up in a car, announces that Jesus is coming soon, and then vanishes? Or did you know there are alligators living in the sewers of New York? They got there because people bought baby alligators at the World's Fair. They brought them home, but when the alligators got too big, they were flushed down the toilet. Well, they didn't die, and now they're huge, living in the sewers, eating cats and rats, and every once in awhile, an unsuspecting sanitation worker. Or maybe you heard the one about "Mikey," the little boy from the cereal commercial in the 1970s. Recently he was eating Pop Rocks candy and drinking a carbonated soda at the same time. This was a deadly combination, and tragically, he died!

As you might suspect, none of the above stories are true, but they're all well known and passed around on a regular basis. The stories and panic about multigenerational satanists are examples of what sociologists refer to as *rumors* or *urban myths*. Rumors involve folklore that people come to believe as true and then share with others. These stories are told in such a way that the next hearer believes the story and passes it on to others. Rumors have a definite quality of entertainment, often told as a scary story. Their exact origins are difficult to discover, but once born, a rumor quickly spreads by word of mouth, written materials, and various media sources. Like a raging grass fire, before you know it, it's everywhere. Mind you, the tellers' intent is not deceitful, for they were told the story by someone else and are simply firm believers who eagerly pass on an exciting bit of news.

Rumors play a very important role in shaping people's beliefs by allowing individuals to take part in a group event, to belong, to be included. A person doesn't simply pass on a rumor, he seeks to convince the listener. Thus rumors convert others to the group's point of view, and the more numbers that can be added to the group, the better. Research has found that the more tightly knit a group is, the greater its vulnerability to rumors because of their shared worldview and a hesitancy to question. You see, by believing in a shared rumor, each member is declaring allegiance to the group. In fact, many groups create powerful, common enemies (real or not) that are viewed as posing an immediate threat. This imminent danger conveniently prevents any questioning of the group's claims, so that skeptics are seen as betraying the group's imperiled cause.

Characteristics of a Rumor

The great enemy of the truth is very often not the lie—
deliberate, contrived and dishonest—
but the myth—persistent, persuasive and unrealistic.
JOHN F. KENNEDY, COMMENCEMENT ADDRESS, JUNE 11, 1962

Expert Sources

Rumors are often revealed by a "well-informed source" who is seen as trustworthy; he is sharing a compelling story he has heard and wants to warn you about some great evil or tell you a fascinating bit of news. The expert source is not the direct actor in the story but the middleman, who is closely connected to the original source and enjoys the special status of being someone "in the know."

Local Details

Often the rumor has local details and proximity to help persuade the hearer of the story's veracity. In the rumor about the praying satanists who are joined by unsuspecting hikers, the setting is always somewhere nearby and experienced by someone whom the speaker knows thirdhand ("My pastor's nephew swears that this happened to him. He and two friends were hiking

out near Bear Canyon when they came across some satanists praying . . .”). The problem is, if you were to check with the nephew
you'd find that it wasn't actually him, he heard it from his professor's wife. And on it goes. A rumor always lacks verifiable details,
like specific dates or who was there, and concrete evidence. When
researchers investigate social rumors they find that details are
changed from town to town, to fit each local community. The
source of the rumor is always just a couple of exchanges away, so
the hearer believes he's getting the "inside scoop."

Confirmations

A group's worldview is an important determinant of which
rumors that group will accept and pass around. Recently liberal
groups circulated a rumor that Snapple Ice Tea was giving its
profits to the Ku Klux Klan. At the time, Snapple was advertising
on a nationally known, conservative radio talk show. It doesn't
take a genius to figure out that, for liberals, their "demons" are
conservatives (whom they associate with the Ku Klux Klan). The
Snapple story had no basis in reality, but it appealed to liberals'
worldview.[20]

Rumors convey information that we want to believe is true.
They appeal to a common worldview and incorporate the demons
that a particular group adheres to. Some feminists have rumors of
patriarchal white males who are highly organized and plotting to
control them. New Agers see the government as covering up evidence for the space aliens. Christians have bought into satanic
rumors, with fantastic tales of conspiracy and deception. What is
shared by these and other groups is a compelling desire to believe
the conspiracy, which disables usual standards of reasoning and
investigation. Rumors seduce us by our desire to believe they are
true. They confirm our previous suspicions and further our
group's righteous cause.

Here's a rumor that made the rounds during the earlier witch-
hunts of the seventeenth century:

> There was a lewd fellow in Belgium who had to do with a cow,
> and the cow soon became pregnant and after some months gave
> birth to a male foetus, which was not a calf but human. There
> were many present who saw it come from its mother's womb,
> and they picked it up from the ground and gave it to a nurse.
> The boy grew up and was baptized and instructed in the
> Christian life, and applied himself seriously to piety and works

of penance for his father; and so came to manhood. But he felt in himself certain bovine propensities, as that of eating grass and chewing the cud. What must be thought of this? Was he not a man? Certainly I believe he was; but I deny his mother was a cow. What then? The devil was aware of his father's sin, and at his pleasure made the cow appear pregnant: he then secretly brought an infant from elsewhere, and so placed it by the laboring cow (which was big only with wind) that it seemed to be born from the cow.[21]

Did you laugh? Think again. For over three hundred years people much like you and me firmly believed and taught these stories. Do you really think the scary stories of satanic panic today are any more valid? Mobile crematoriums, hundreds of thousands of murders (but no bodies, or for that matter no missing thousands), zero evidence for multigenerational satanists, dish detergent with the Mark of the Beast on its label.

"Those who do not remember the past are condemned to relive it," said George Santayana. The current satanic panic being experienced needs to be seen within a historical context. In the 1980s and '90s, we are bearing witness to the rebirth of the witch-hunts. Mind you, this is not *like* the witch-hunts, it literally *is* the witch-hunts, the next cycle, the real McCoy. With stunning accuracy, today's inquisitors have reintroduced the panic of centuries ago and, once again, thousands are being destroyed in its wake.

Points to Remember

✓ Four types of satanists have been identified: *dabblers, self-styled, religious,* and *multigenerational.*

✓ It is the multigenerational satanists who represent the controversy for the Christian community and law enforcement. In over twelve thousand cases of alleged SRA, not a single case related to well-organized satanic rings was shown to be true.

✓ Stories of multigenerational satanists are based on *rumors* (*urban myths*) that appeal to the Christian belief system, have expert sources, local details, and lack direct confirmation. The current False Memory Crisis replicates earlier panics in which rumors fueled witch-hunts and societal hysterias.

6

What's Your Sign?

It is the nature of an hypothesis, when once a man has conceived it, that it assimilates every thing to itself as proper nourishment, and, from the first moment of your begetting it, it generally grows the stronger by every thing you see, hear, read, or understand.
LAURENCE STERNE, TRISTRAM SHANDY, 1759–67

I met Amy at a conference in Texas where I was lecturing on the False Memory Crisis. Her beautiful, quiet smile camouflaged the tremendous torture she had endured in her years of regression therapy. Frightened, her voice quivering, but with a quiet dignity and honesty she discussed her story with several dozen families and professionals, all crowded into a conference room. I noticed the dozens of scars running up and down her arms, reminders of the many times she had cut her wrists in desperate attempts to end her pain. In beginning her story, she showed us a beautiful diamond ring she was wearing. "It sparkled and sang in my cupped palm. The ring had laid nestled in the cotton-filled box for over two years. My mother's anniversary ring from long ago, to be presented to me, her daughter, on my twenty-first birthday. But I was nowhere to be found on that birthday. I had gotten sucked up into a frightful whirlwind, dragging everyone else with me through the pit. The glint from the diamond represents the spark of hope which gleamed through the dark valley of the shadow of death through which my family has groped. . . .

"Although I grew up in a nice home, with nice things, we had not been a happy family. My father was a highly respected obstetrician, and my mother was an incredible artist and housewife. Yet, my brother was schizophrenic and has struggled with it since I can remember. My mother suffers from multiple sclerosis and depression. My father seemed domineering and resentful, and I tried very hard to be the 'perfect child,' holding the facade together. By my senior year in high school, I hated myself for being imperfect and hated my family for the same reason. I talked to no one. At last I had to be hospitalized for anorexia. I was the perfect patient. I worked hard, gained ten pounds, had some family sessions, and was then released. Unfortunately, my problems quickly reappeared.

"Back in college, I was once again battling unrealistic expectations, and after three semesters I again desperately needed help. Some school counselors referred me to a hospital, where I was quickly admitted for bulimia. My social worker was a bitter and paranoid woman, who insisted that my father abused me and that I needed to 'unpry' these memories to have any chance of getting better. I wanted more than anything to be the perfect patient once again, and I plunged right in. I worked day and night to find those memories, and my anxiety rose to unbearable levels. I kept on, though, motivated by the encouraging, 'Amy, you're doing great, you're working so hard!' Two-and-a-half months later they were still telling me this and I was an emotional wreck, acting self-destructive and suicidal. My parents, after paying eighty thousand dollars, said that I could only have a few more weeks of inpatient care. The doctors indicated that this showed lack of cooperation, support, and interest in my behalf. My social worker told me that it showed my parents had something to hide.

"When my insurance was reinstated three months later, I was readmitted. At this time they opened the new 'dissociative disorders unit,' which I read made over fifteen thousand dollars a day. There were about nine of us, and all of the women were between the ages of twenty and fifty. Many had husbands and children. If our insurance was good, we were told we should expect to stay for at least six months. All I can say is, thank goodness I had crummy insurance!

"I say this because life on this unit was a nightmare. I could go on for hours about the events that took place on this unit, and they are not different from the experiences of most FMS [False Memory Syndrome] victims. Suffice to say that through daily hypnosis, abreaction sessions in leather restraints, psychodrama, and dissociative exercises, my memories transformed over time into horrific scenes of torture, pornography, satanic rituals, and murder. Every remote, even happy, memory I had from childhood became some elaborate traumatic experience. To this day when I see pictures of me as a young girl, I feel an ache in my heart. Not because I believe any of the false memories, but [because] my real memories have become so tainted. It was as if the doctors, intentionally or not, took that innocent little girl and ripped her apart.

"In the fall of 1990 I told my parents I never wanted to see them again. This was devastating and totally unexpected for them. From that point on, most attempts on their part to try to help me or communicate with me were seen as an attempt to control or manipulate me, and I would not tolerate it.

"My work with the hospital ended when my insurance ran out. I continued to see my doctor and therapist. This therapy became too consuming and even too dangerous to continue. I started to become paranoid, believing there were cult members out to get me, and I struggled daily with over a dozen fabricated personalities. I was tired and had to stop.

"Over a very gradual process, I started to question my memories. I actually had always questioned them, several times a day, in fact, but I was always rebutted, and told that, first, there's no way to fabricate memories with such emotion and clarity, and second, even if I could make such violent and gory stuff up, that would mean that I was *really* psychotic and demented. This is what hooked me for so long, because even when the memories seemed totally preposterous, I had to believe that I couldn't have just created them in my own mind. I was always seen as such a nice, sweet girl. I cared deeply for all living things. I did volunteer work every chance I got. In fact, it was continuous volunteer work that kept me going through this whole ordeal. How could someone like that do all this to her own parents?

"I started to realize that there was no proof for any of my allegations. In fact, there was only monumental conflicting evidence. I also realized that these memories weren't really memories, but mere stories concocted in the presence of the hospital staff. I hoped that I could just heal, that the flashbacks and images would subside. But they didn't. They kept recurring with the same anger, fear, and pain over and over again.

"This is where the False Memory Foundation came in. In August of 1993, I came across an article describing a patient's experiences at the same hospital and [how she] recanted her memories. The descriptions were just too similar to be a coincidence. The article also stated that the dissociative unit had been investigated and closed down, for it was found that the patients' treatment was unethical. This article exhilarated me, angered and depressed me, relieved and dumbfounded me. I immediately made a copy and wrote on the side, 'I can't tell you how sorry I am.' I mailed this to my parents just to let them know that I truly was sorry. I never expected to hear from them. I had no idea that they knew about FMS. I assumed I had ruined any chance of ever being a part of my family again. Well, my parents received it less than twenty-four hours later. Nothing I have ever mailed [from] four hundred miles away arrived so promptly!

"My parents called that evening. The conversation was very tense. I don't even remember what was said. I just remember the relief and excitement in my mother's voice. The next few months were extremely emotional as we discussed reuniting. My paternal grandparents had died during the ordeal, but my maternal grandparents were anxious to see me. With Laura Pasley's [another retractor] help, my mother and I reunited in October on the *Donahue* show, and I met with my grandmother backstage. We all flew back to see the rest of my family. It was wonderful and totally exhausting. I cried that night, and my mother stayed with me and hugged me. I never before felt so close to her.

"It has taken me a while to train myself not to dissociate, contemplate suicide, or use the dysfunctional coping skills I learned while in the hospital. I recently learned something interesting. My dissociative episodes derived from fits of queasiness, shaking, nausea, and fatigue. This was translated into anxiety, which the doctors indicated was due to some unknown secret trying to surface. I still, to this day, have these episodes, although I have learned not to dissociate during them. I saw another doctor and had some blood work done and have discovered that those 'panic attacks' are a result of being hypoglycemic!

"I have moved back to be close to my family again. My grandparents helped me pay off my remaining debt, so I could move sooner. I have been free of my bulimia for almost a year. I struggle daily with depression, much of which is likely rooted in the craziness of the past few years. I have had to rely greatly on my parents through this time for support and reassurance as I face the life I left five years ago. I missed a lot in those years, and I grieve over that. If one good thing has come out of all of this, it is a newfound appreciation of my family, and we have all gained an awareness and respect for each other's thoughts and feelings."[1]

Reading the Signs

Regression literature always contains lists of symptoms that regressionists use to confirm that someone has repressed memories of trauma. One of the most common is from E. Sue Blume's book, *Secret Survivors*. Blume offers thirty-five categories, with over 180 "symptoms" a person can read through to discover if he or she has repressed memories. A few of them are: fearing the dark, having nightmares, not liking your body, having sponta-neous vaginal infections, getting headaches, arthritis, wearing lots of clothes, preferring privacy when using the bathroom, being scared of different things, needing to be invisible, not being funny, doing what others want, blocking out memories between the first and twelfth years of life, being in denial, not enjoying sex, not lik-ing gynecological exams, avoiding mirrors, avoiding making noises, or stealing things.[2]

Whew! Take a breath.

You might also find yourself feeling guilty, shameful, valueless, worthless, abandoned, different, unhappy, crazy, or wanting to change your name. You might abuse drugs or not abuse drugs, think you're perfectly good or perfectly bad, have constant anger or don't get angry, can't trust others or trust too much, take too many risks or don't take risks, are controlling or fear losing con-trol, feel real or feel unreal, don't like particular sex acts or like particular sex acts, are seductive or not interested in sex, are sexu-ally aggressive or not, or your relationships are ambivalent or they're conflicted.[3]

The list goes on for over 180 colorful, exotic items and the author lets the reader know that her list will never be complete! My question is: How did you do on her list? It literally predicts that everyone alive is the victim of abuse. With heavy feminist themes, Blume offers her indicators of "hidden abuse" based on clinical observations and anecdotal stories, without any scientific validation. You might laugh at the absurdity, but imagine going to a therapist when you're lonely and depressed. Your guard is down and you're desperate for answers. Your new therapist hands you Blume's list. Think you'd be influenced by it? Thousands have been.

Quotes emblazoned on her book cover proclaim the virtues of this "symptoms checklist." Gloria Steinem, the feminist leader, proclaims that Blume's list "explores the constellation of symp-toms that result from a crime too cruel for mind and memory to face. This book, like the truth it helps to uncover, can set millions free."[4] Elisabeth Kubler-Ross, a leader in grief and loss research, offers, "A resource of excellent caliber. . . . Highly recommended for those who suspect that they are unconscious survivors of abuse and especially for therapists to dig into the darkest shadow part of human existence."[5] Claudia Black, one of the founders of the vic-tims' movement, describes the book as "powerful and compre-hensive. *Secret Survivors* is a major contribution to understanding the issues that confront incest survivors. It must be read by all."[6] These "experts" are willing to promote the crude, magical thinking of Blume's list without a shred of scientific validity.

"Alice," a retractor from regression therapy, stated: "It's horrible brainwashing—you're paranoid of everything. Any problems I was having in my life were interpreted by my therapists as signs of childhood sexual abuse. I got to the point where I couldn't tell real from unreal. The psychotherapist told me point-blank he knew I was sexually abused the second time he met me because I had a problem with control issues."[7] Another retractor reported her therapist's conclusions: "This must have happened to you because you have the symptoms, therefore if you can't remember the abuse we may need to increase your dosage or change drugs."[8] "Christine," also a retractor, commented, "When I questioned them, the therapist would reinforce the check list in Sue Blume's book *Secret Survivors*, she would tell me, 'You checked off 33 of the 35 indicators, how could this possibly be wrong? Professionals recognize this as being gospel truth.'"[9]

Here's a similar list of symptoms I came across in a recent study. The results were proclaimed in newspapers throughout the United States. See if you can figure out what the symptoms indicate.

- Waking up paralyzed with the sense of a strange presence in the room
- Lost periods of time
- The experience of flying through the air without knowing how or why
- Seeing unusual lights or balls of light in a room
- Discovering puzzling scars on your body without knowing how they got there. [10]

Some additional symptoms include anxiety, depression, phobias, or a pattern of frightening dreams, memory gaps, symptoms consistent with PTSD, gynecological problems, and false pregnancies.[11] John Mack, professor of psychiatry at Harvard Medical School, also provides a list of symptoms for the same trauma: fears of the dark, nightmares, other fears, phobic symptoms, missing time episodes, small cuts, scars, odd red spots.[12]

Have you figured it out? These are indicators for space alien abductions. Using these "symptoms," a national Roper survey proclaimed that two out of every hundred people have been space-alien abducted, but do not recall the experience. If you're wondering, that makes over one hundred million abductions worldwide.[13]

Or how about this list: "phobias, panic attacks, recurrent nightmares, unexplained fears, obesity, repeated destructive relationships, physical pain and illness." Theses are symptoms of hidden traumas that have occurred in *prior* lives.[14]

There's more. A recovery book describes signs of satanic ritualistic abuse: Physical disorders include seizures, liver malfunctions, adrenal gland problems, problems with digestion, bladder/kidney infections, skin irritations, headaches, asthma, being overweight, vaginal infections, sexually transmitted diseases, unusual scars, numbing in different parts of the body, chronic pain. Nervous and phobic symptoms include exaggerated startle response, hypervigilance, panic attacks, allergies, aversion to drinking water, multiple psychiatric hospitalizations, claustrophobia, sense of impending doom, fear of one's birthday, intense paranoia, fears/phobias, hypochondriasis, general sense of terror, fear of abandonment.

Psychological disorders include self-mutilation, history of suicide attempts, alcoholism or other drug abuse, eating disorders, mood swings, sexual problems, compulsive washing of the genitals, bed-wetting as a child, MPD, dissociative disorder, paranoid schizophrenic, borderline personality, manic/depression, bipolar, psychotic disorder, addictive orders, depersonalization disorder, PTSD, lying, sleep disorders, hallucinations, or hearing voices, depression.[15]

Then there's the varied assortment of indicators, which include fluctuation in behaviors and skills, driving fast, being in physically dangerous locations, being fascinated by the supernatural, childhood amnesia, being easily induced into a trance state, switching therapists frequently, crying or laughing, being drawn to or repulsed by occult themes, being convinced one is possessed or evil, having a belief that one is controlled by something or someone outside of him- or herself, having imaginary friends as a child or adult, having a sense of unreality, black-and-white thinking, flat feelings, or unusual behaviors.[16]

Are you getting my point? National "trauma experts" pulled together a fantastic array of symptoms they felt were indicators of whichever particular trauma they believed was in their clients. There are over nine hundred "symptoms" that have been identified in regression literature that supposedly point to a history of abuse. But not a single symptom has been scientifically validated as an actual indicator of repressed memories.[17] The American Psychological Association agrees: "There is no single set of symptoms which automatically means that a person was a victim of childhood abuse."[18] These imaginative lists have no basis in reality but instead are based on the conclusions that the regressionist wants the client to reach. In scientific terms, the symptoms lack *discriminate validity*, that is, they don't differentiate between numerous psychological and personality disorders or normalcy. What is amazing is the amount of regard these lists are given by regressionists and "survivors," who are willing to risk health, safety, and their connection to reality by believing these are legitimate.

Interestingly, as similar as the lists are, it is up to the regressionist to determine which kind of trauma you've forgotten. If the regressionist specializes in SRA, then the symptoms always point to satanic traumas; if the regressionist is a UFO specialist, then the same list is indicative of space alien trauma. Sigmund Freud explained, "If the first-discovered scene is unsatisfactory, we tell our patient that this experience explains nothing, but that behind it there must be hidden a more significant, earlier, experience. . . . A continuation of the analysis then leads in every instance to the reproduction of new scenes of the character we expect."[19] Modern-day regressionists closely follow Freud's lead, interrogating patients until they create images in keeping with what the regressionist expects: a hidden history of sexual, ritual, space alien, or past-lives trauma. If the results were not as devastating to the lives of clients and their families, these lists could be viewed as comical. In reality, their function is to initiate a belief system in a vulnerable client, who can later be manipulated through the use of hypnotic techniques to come to believe the fantastic. Though a therapist may be well meaning, he can still do tremendous harm.

The idea of special signs or symptoms pointing toward an evildoer's guilt or an innocent person's victimization isn't new. As we noted in the last chapter, the satanic panic we are currently experiencing is a repeated cycle of the witch-hunts that occurred for over three hundred years in Europe. At that time a number of symptoms "proving" that someone was afflicted by a witch were also developed, without scientific or legal validation. The lists were equally as far-fetched, including eating disorders, purging, digestion problems, stomach tightness, urinary problems, neck pain, headaches, heart difficulties, body swelling, sudden out-bursts, lethargy, depression, pain in the limbs, ulcers, withdraw-ing behaviors, skin discoloration, eye problems, and panic attacks.[20]

The bottom line: There is no list of symptoms *anywhere* that has been scientifically shown to be a reliable indicator of hidden abuse. In the light of day, these lists are revealed as primitive, superstitious psychobabble which have destroyed the lives of thousands.

Alternative Questions

Rossell Robbins reports on a prosecutorial method called *alternative questions* used during the witch-hunts. These were designed in such a way that every answer was indicative of guilt:

QUESTION: Is the accused in bad repute?

CONCLUSION: If so, she is a witch. If not, she is undoubtedly a witch, for witches always seek to be well thought of.

QUESTION: Is the accused frightened?

CONCLUSION: If so, she is a witch. If not, she is undoubtedly a witch.

QUESTION: Does the accused admit guilt?

CONCLUSION: If so, she is a witch. If not, she is undoubtedly a witch, for witches always represent themselves as innocent.[21]

Robbins noted, "Once an [idea] has obsessed a person, a group, or a nation, then every word and deed, no matter how disparate or irrelevant, serves to confirm the mania."[22] Those words, writ-ten in 1960 and referring to deeds which occurred hundreds of years ago, are hauntingly appropriate today. When fantasies of abuse are turned into criminal proof, the presumption is guilt, not innocence.

In the modern courtroom, in the media, and in the opinions of family and friends, the situation is similar to the witch trials. For example:

QUESTION: Does the accused seem to be a nice person?
CONCLUSION: If so, he is undoubtedly a perpetrator, for perpetrators always seek to be well thought of. If not, he is a perpetrator.

QUESTION: Is the accused frightened?
CONCLUSION: If so, he is guilty. If not, he is undoubtedly guilty.

QUESTION: Does the accused admit guilt?
CONCLUSION: If so, he is a perpetrator. If not, he is undoubtedly a perpetrator, for perpetrators always represent themselves as innocent. He must be in denial!

This style of "alternate questions" is reflected in Blume's "either/or" questions (drug abuse or no drug use, perfectionism or nonperfectionism, constant anger or lack of anger, etc.). Professional illusionists refer to this as "magician's choice." No matter which way a person answers, the regressionist will take the client to the predetermined conclusion. The American Psychiatric Association warns, "There is no uniform (profile) or other method to accurately distinguish those who have sexually abused children from those who have not."[23]

Details of Accounts

A common argument I heard for repression is that "People's details of recovered memories are similar, so this proves they must be valid." SRA believers will point to common details of bells, candles, black robes, and ritual practices that they "recover" in their hypnotic fantasies. UFO believers note that there are universal descriptions of the aliens, medical examinations, and shapes of their spacecrafts. Pointing to similarities in recovered memory reports is nothing new. When Freud was arguing for repression, he told his colleagues, "There is the uniformity which they exhibit in certain details, which is a necessary consequence if the preconditions of these experiences are always of the same kind, but which would otherwise lead us to believe that there were secret understandings between the various patients."[24]

We can go back even further. In justifying torture and murder, the witch-hunters argued that uniformity of detail proved that the accused were guilty:

With so much agreement and conformity between the different cases, that the most ignorant persons convicted of this crime have spoken to the same circumstances, and in nearly the same words, as the most celebrated authors who have written about it. All of which may be easily proved to your majesty's satisfaction by the records of various trials before your parliaments.[25]

The witch-hunters of three hundred years ago and the regressionists of today share a common misconception. They assume that the similarity in details proves the accusations, but they fail to see that it is they themselves who create the uniform reports through their own teachings, media influence, recovery groups, seminars, and readings. In science we call this a *contagion effect.*

Bob and Gretchen Passantino demonstrate how details of a hysteria can be subtly passed along. A therapist had been doing regression therapy on a fifty-two-year-old client, who spontaneously recovered childhood memories of being a little girl living in the Southwest during World War II. She "remembered" being abducted to Rome by a group of satanists, where she says she was repeatedly raped by the Pope. She maintained that this had occurred on several occasions and her parents had no knowledge of these events! Mind you, this client claims that she was flown by propeller airplane across the United States, across the Atlantic, through war-time Europe for sexual flings with the Pope and both she and her parents had no knowledge of her abduction and violent rapes.

But wait! There's more! This same therapist had another client whom he was treating at the time. This second client *also* recovered memories of being abducted by satanists to Rome, where she was raped by the Pope. Remember, this was a spontaneous disclosure—the two clients didn't know each other, and this was not a story that had been published anywhere. This means that their stories were not contaminated by outside sources, they were "authentic."

Very excited, the therapist contacted the Passantinos and declared that he had discovered proof of the existence of multigenerational satanists. Two clients, with no relationship to one another, produced the same detailed repressed memories. But the Passantinos were able to help the therapist understand that the two clients actually shared something in common—each had the same therapist. He had given both of them the same material to read and coached them in the same direction. Most importantly, the women actually had contact in an informal setting—the waiting room. Occasionally they had back-to-back appointments, so while he was finishing his notes from the first client, the two women were in the waiting room sharing their experiences. Presto! With that subtle interaction both were able to create the same traumatic fantasies.[26]

What this story illustrates is that, as in the development of rumors, individuals do not have to be in direct contact in order to acquire common information. The recovery community is particularly vulnerable to rumors because of the multiple, interconnected communication and education networks shared by therapists and clients. Studies of group processes show that at its start members are not saying the same thing, but as time progresses, the group becomes more alike in its beliefs. Common readings, zealous leaders, and group members will literally teach the new convert how to develop traumatic fantasies with similar themes and details.

Points to Remember

✔ *Regression literature* always contains imaginative lists of "symptoms" for whatever trauma it's promoting. These lists have no scientific basis and lack *discriminate validity*.

✔ The "symptoms" for repressed incest, SRA, past lives, and alien abductions are quite similar—the conclusion of which alleged trauma the patient suffers from is based on the treating therapist's bias.

✔ *Alternative questions* are a typical feature of regression symptoms lists. It sets up a "double bind" in which either response by the client is indicative of repressed trauma.

✔ *Contagion effect* occurs when a client's hypnotic images are influenced by regression teachings, media influence, recovery groups, seminars, and readings. The subsequent similarity of details in hypnotic accounts is misread as evidence of validity, when it actually points back to common sources of contagion that vulnerable clients are being exposed to.

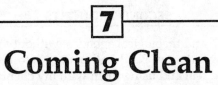

7

Coming Clean

*A man should never be ashamed to own he has been in the wrong,
which is but saying, in other words, that he is wiser today than he
was yesterday.*

JONATHAN SWIFT, *THOUGHTS ON VARIOUS SUBJECTS*, 1711

I was finding that one by one, the assumptions I had so fervently believed and taught were falling apart under closer inspection.

- The theory of repressed memory was just that, a *theory* which Freud created and later rejected. Despite one hundred years of research, there still was no scientific evidence confirming its reality. When we know that a traumatic event has occurred, the exact opposite happens—people are plagued by recurrent memories of their trauma, as in instances of post-traumatic stress disorder.

- Even if there were valid cases of repression, the techniques used in regressionism had not been demonstrated to actually unlock repressed events. In fact, they created highly delusional states of mind in which clients were vulnerable to suggestion and vivid fantasies.

- Of the thousands of hypnotic fantasies of incest, SRA, past lives, and space aliens, I knew that some considerable portion was false. But neither I nor any of my regression colleagues were doing anything to account for false positives.

- The stories of multigenerational satanists were without any scientific or law-enforcement evidence. These stories, described by highly suggestible and mentally disturbed individuals, were far from reliable and in over twelve thousand cases failed to be confirmed as real. The belief in multigenerational satanists reflected a strong urban mythology that had deeply entrenched itself within the Christian community.

- There were no such thing as "symptoms" of forgotten abuse. These lists were developed by individuals with extreme political, social, and theological agendas, without any reference to scientific validation. But I had bought into them, mistaking them to be real and using them with my clients.

In 1992, my pursuit of truth was beginning to lead me away from my regression involvement and back to common sense and the scientific discipline of psychology in which I had trained for so many years. It was during this time of questioning that I learned of the newly formed *False Memory Syndrome Foundation*, headquartered in Philadelphia. This organization represented the coming together of professionals, researchers, and clinicians from psychiatry, psychology, social work, law, and education from across the nation who were awakening to the False Memory Crisis. With a focus on memory, professional standards, suggestibility, and hypnosis, experts provided me with desperately needed information. I quickly discovered that I was not alone in my growing doubts; they too had borne witness to the devastating aftermath of the regression movement and had begun to question its practices. Having been locked inside a closed regression belief system, I finally experienced the opportunity to hear a different perspective, one which helped confirm my growing doubts.

False Memory Syndrome

It's been referred to as *decade-delayed disclosure, pseudomemories,* and *confabulation*. But *false memory syndrome* (FMS) is the most popular name that has been given to the phenomenon in which a person experiences vivid fantasies of traumatic events, fantasies which they have come to believe are real. Unlike the theory of repression, false memories are a well-established and documented phenomenon in research literature. We reviewed some of this research in Chapter 4. But common sense also points to the reality of false memories. The New Hampshire Supreme Court noted:

> It must be acknowledged that "false" memories do occur. This is known by the existence of cases in which it is impossible that the events remembered occurred, such as in cases of remembered alien abductions. A further indication of the potential for false memories are the recantation of a growing number of those who once claimed recovered memories.[1]

As the court pointed out, of the thousands of reports of incest, satanic ritual abuse, space alien abductions, and prior lives, it stands to reason that at least some portion of these hypnotic images are false.

Dr. John Kihlstrom, a cognitive psychologist and professor at Yale University, provides an excellent definition of FMS:

> False Memory Syndrome—a condition in which a person's identity and interpersonal relationships are centered around a memory of traumatic experience which is objectively false but in which the person strongly believes. Note that the syndrome is not characterized by false memories as such. We all have memories that are inaccurate. Rather, the syndrome may be diagnosed when the memory is so deeply ingrained that it orients the individual's entire personality and lifestyle, in turn disrupting all sorts of other adaptive behaviors. The analogy to personality disorder is intentional. False memory syndrome is especially destructive because the person assiduously avoids confrontation with any evidence that might challenge the memory. Thus it takes on a life of its own, encapsulated and resistant to correction. The person may become so focused on the memory that he or she may be effectively distracted from coping with the real problems in his or her life.[2]

Dr. Kihlstrom points out several important aspects of FMS. One is that a person's identity and relationships become centered around her hypnotic images. Like a convert to a new religion, the patient's pursuit and exploration of these images becomes all-consuming. Parenting of children, working, maintaining a good marriage, being active in church—all of these obligations quickly take a backseat to the convert's new pursuit. The only thing she reads or talks about is repression. Therapy, group sessions, and readings continue to increase, and regressionism insidiously becomes her entire world. In this new religion, the god of regressionism is a fierce taskmaster, demanding 110 percent of her devotion and servitude.

A second aspect that Dr. Kihlstrom points out is that the person avoids any contradictory evidence that might prove the images false. A relationship with anyone who is not completely supportive and believing is terminated. Research, books, and media programs explaining the phenomenon of false memories are seen as "propaganda" fostered by perpetrators and those who are still "in denial" about space aliens, prior lives, incest, and so on. Regressionism is designed as a lifelong pursuit.

The Big Picture

What about this word, *syndrome*, referring to a pattern of symptoms that point toward a possible disease or condition? Those studying false memory *syndrome* seek to identify the pattern that is emerging for clients who are involved in regression therapy. What's been discovered so far? Research through the FMS Foundation reveals some interesting demographics. The people experiencing hypnotic images are most often:[3]

- Caucasian (97 percent)
- Female (92 percent)
- Young (81 percent are aged twenty to thirty-nine)
- Middle- to upper-class (92 percent)
- Highly educated and high-achieving (59 percent have college degrees as compared to 17 percent in the general population).[4]

Consider what these observations tell us. We know that actual child abuse is found in every spectrum of society. When I was working with abused children through Child Protective Services, I encountered families and victims in every socioeconomic class, from every walk of life. In sharp contrast, those claiming recovered traumatic memories are predominately white, young females who are well educated and in the middle- to upper-class. Why aren't we seeing minorities, older, less-educated or lower-middle-class people experiencing recovered memories? Basically, they're not the ones in therapy. This gives us an important clue to the origins of the False Memory Crisis, as we'll discover in the next two chapters.

What is it that people with traumatic hypnotic images describe?

- 68 percent of alleged abuse is supposed to have begun before the age of four. (Keep in mind that memory prior to age four is very unreliable.)
- The most common length of repression is thirty to forty years.
- 13 percent of the allegations involve one or two traumatic episodes. But 53 percent report multiple episodes of trauma (robust repression).

- In the allegations, 22 percent include accusations of rape and 18 percent include satanic ritual abuse themes.[5]

Caution: Deadly Therapy Ahead

Washington State allows individuals to receive treatment under the Crime Victims Act, including those who claim repressed memories of childhood abuse. Recently the Washington Department of Labor and Industries completed a preliminary study to see how effective regression therapy has been. A researcher randomly selected thirty cases to investigate. Her findings are compelling:[6]

- 97 percent of the patients were women.
- 97 percent were Caucasian.
- 87 percent received their first "memories" of abuse while in therapy.
- The average age of the first "recalled" abuse was 7 *months* of age.
- 100 percent were still in therapy three years after the first "memory" (60 percent were still in therapy five after years after their first "memory").
- Prior to recovered memory therapy only 10 percent exhibited suicidal ideation or attempts, after therapy began this jumped up to 67 percent.
- Prior to therapy 10 percent had been hospitalized, after therapy this expanded to 37 percent.
- Prior to therapy only 3 percent had engaged in self-mutilation, after therapy this grew to 27 percent.
- Prior to therapy 83 percent were employed, after therapy only 10 percent were still employed.
- Prior to therapy 77 percent were married. Three years later 48 percent were separated or divorced.
- After therapy began 23 percent had lost custody of their children.
- After therapy began 100 percent were estranged from their extended family.
- The average cost for the Crime Victim Compensation Program to pay for treatment of patients that *did not* involve recovered memories was $2,672. The average cost for recovered memory therapy was dramatically higher: $12,296 (more than four-and-a-half times the normal cost).

The implications are clear. Regressionism is a massively expensive "therapy" in which patients get worse, dramatically worse, with no end or recovery in sight. Imagine if regressionism were pills in a bottle sitting on the shelf at your local pharmacy. Based on the clearly destructive results of these "pills" the Food and Drug Administration would have them off the shelf yesterday. But the field of psychology lacks any kind of independent safety board. The exotic, deadly claims of regressionists go unchecked, destroying thousands in their wake. Even if there are actual cases of repression, we now know that the proposed "cure" of regression therapies is often deadlier than the disease.

What False Memory Syndrome Is Not

In understanding what the false memory syndrome *is*, it is also important to understand what it is *not*. As we discussed, false memory syndrome occurs when a person experiences hypnotic images which are partially or completely fictional. FMS is by no means a denial of the fact that actual child abuse occurs and does not question the reality of free standing memories of abuse. What come into question are hypnotic images of abuse that a person claims to have remembered after a period of decades or centuries. At best, these images may reflect a real event, a complete fantasy, or some distorted combination of the two extremes. Those who are critiquing regressionism maintain a healthy balance in recognizing the tragedy of childhood abuse and the reality of the False Memory Crisis.

The Families

With research and a caring skepticism, the FMS Foundation is seeking to better understand the regression movement and educate other professionals and the general public about the growing crisis. Central to its mission is reaching out to thousands of families who have been devastated by repressed memory accusations from their children. As of June 1996, more than seventeen thousand families have identified themselves as victims of FMS and have contacted the Foundation. What exactly do these families look like? A 1993 survey showed that 90 percent of them were middle- to upper-class at the time the accusing child was growing up.[7] They have stable marriages, with 71 percent of the parents still married, and of those, 88 percent have been married over thirty years.[8] They tend to be very involved in their faith, with 81 percent identifying themselves as active Christians.[9] Interestingly, families who described themselves as very active in their faith are more likely to be accused of being multigenerational satanists.[10]

Fifty-one percent of the time the father is the only one accused. The mother is accused of active participation in the abuse (alone and/or with her spouse) 42 percent of the time.[11] Two-thirds (67 percent) of parents have no contact with their accusing child and 39 percent have lost contact with their grandchildren.[12] Also, two-thirds (66 percent) of the parents have never met their child's treating therapist, and 41 percent of them were served a "confrontation letter" informing them that they were guilty of child abuse and other crimes.[13] Seventy-one percent of the siblings do not believe the accusing child's reports.[14]

Stop for a second and feel what I've just described. These are more than just numbers on a page. These figures reflect the torture and destruction of thousands of lives and families. Without opportunity to defend themselves, people's reputations and families have been wiped out based on the whim of a hypnotic fantasy. The injustice that we as a society have engaged in is enormous.

I was starting to realize that I had been an integral part of this injustice. I had believed my clients who were making the accusations, but I wasn't allowing the accused, the parents and siblings, to be a part of their own trial and conviction. I had learned that a local chapter of the FMS Foundation had just been formed in the Phoenix area. Skeptical and guarded, I decided to attend their next meeting, convinced that I would encounter a room full of pedophiles and satanists. I couldn't have been more wrong. Here were families that represented the very heart of the American family. They had lived productive lives, raised their children, worked in their professions. Despite their various backgrounds, each shared a common experience. Their grown children had gone into therapy, and from there, with little warning, the nightmare had begun. The horrifying accusations and hateful letters that followed had left these parents devastated and confused, desperately looking for answers.

From the start, the families were very suspicious of my presence. I was the first psychologist who had attended their meetings. For them I represented the enemy, one of the professionals that had devoured their children. They weren't far off in their suspicions. Some of their children were clients I worked with in therapy. Incredibly, the families and I were able let down our guard and talk. I let them know about my involvement in regressionism and my growing doubts. Slowly, these tender, gray-haired elders began to reveal to me their tremendous pain and despair. "Helen's" story was typical. As she talked, her eyes burnt brilliant with an unwavering faith in Christ. A mother and grandmother, she has spent decades serving God in a number of ministries. I was impressed with the depth and quality of faith that I sensed in her.

"Six very long years ago, my husband and I were accused by our youngest daughter, who was in her thirties, of satanic ritual abuse, along with many other accusations that were just horrible: killing babies, having our six children doing these acts of horror, poking out babies' eyes with knives. She said that we used to take animals, you know, dogs and cats, and sacrifice them, cook them on the backyard grill, and then eat them. She says one night we ordered a pizza, when the delivery boy came to our door, we enticed him into our home, killed him, barbecued him on the outside grill, and then ate him.

"I don't know why my daughter began therapy. She went to two Christian counselors who were reputed in our community to be satanic ritual abuse and multiple-personality disorder experts, although they only had high-school educations. They felt that their therapy was a 'new working of the Holy Spirit,' and He was their guide in this bold form of 'healing.' Anyway, early in therapy, these counselors convinced my daughter that she was sexually abused as a child, that her family were members of a satanic cult, and though they had never met me, that I was suffering from a multiple-personality disorder. They tried to involve my other adult children in these 'recovered memories,' and when they refused to participate, the list of accused grew to include them as well. Sisters and brothers, neighbors, friends, other family members, and finally church members—as time passed, the list of supposed satanists just kept expanding.

"During the early stages of therapy, my daughter's behavior was very erratic. One moment she would be hugging and kissing me, and the next she would seem very distant. There was a time when my oldest daughter, Becky, and her three children were invited to one of her sister's 'therapy sessions.' It lasted two nights and three days. They would not allow Becky to shower, be alone, even to go to the bathroom. In order to obtain evidence for the police, they videotaped an interview session with the children, asking them about the cult activities of their grandparents. The session lasted until midnight, although the youngest was only three years old. After three days, Becky realized that things weren't right, but they wouldn't let her leave. She managed to break away to a phone and call 911. One man grabbed her to stop her, and the therapist took the phone away and told the operator that 'things were under control,' but the police came anyway. My daughter was taken to the hospital in an ambulance, where she was treated for exhaustion.

"We didn't know what was going on until some people from church came up and told me about our youngest's insinuations. It was only my faith in God that took us through this. There were times when no one would get near us and the pews around us were empty. I remember that once I attended a women's meeting at the church; it was packed. I sat alone at a table set for eight. Our pastor was very wise and discerning, and he saw this as an attack from the enemy on the family. He had three different meetings discussing our situation with the church and spoke about the gossip directly from the pulpit. He had no fear. He recognized that we were all victims. He took the situation to the board, had us thoroughly investigated, went down to the counseling center, spoke to the people who were involved, and to our son-in-law and daughter. I praise God for this man who stood by us while we were waiting to be vindicated by the police.

"It took three or four years for church members, who were confused by the lies and didn't know what to believe, to ask forgiveness for their attitudes toward us. Even though a piece of our lives is gone, there has been growth in the Lord. We have gained understanding for others who are going through their own pain, and, strangely enough, we have seen God's grace and peace through all of this."

Another couple, "Tom" and "Alice," confided, "We were just getting up, starting our morning routine. You know, sipping coffee and reading the paper. Suddenly there was this pounding at the door. Tom went to see who it was and there was a swarm of police, with search warrants and guns drawn. Our grown daughter and two of her childhood friends had accused us of masterminding the deadly rituals of a cult, saying we had murdered innocent men and children as human sacrifices. The police ordered us to sit on the couch and spent five hours searching for evidence. We were so shocked and confused. Then the phone rang. Various families, our lifetime friends, were calling to tell us that the police had also stormed their homes and were scouring for clues. The police even went so far as to dig up backyards, looking for bodies. Of course the police found nothing. But they refuse to close the case. They still think we did these horrible things."

"Sam" and "Lucy," both in their eighties, described their shock as they were suddenly accused by their daughter, Rachel, of killing three small children in a sleepy Idaho town nearly forty years earlier. Her images of the murders had come back to her during the course of therapy. Rachel had contacted the sheriff in that area, who dismissed her allegations, "Lady, we have no record of any children being murdered in this town in this century. Certainly if three children had been murdered, we would have known about it." Rachel's husband begged her to get decent psychological help, but she refused. Their marriage eventually broke up under the strain of her continued involvement in regressionism. Rachel lost her job and was now, amazingly, looking to her bewildered parents as her only means of financial support. The rest of the family believed in the parents' innocence and dismissed the charges as a bizarre delusion. But Rachel still clung to her story.

On and on the stories went, each one more tragic and obscene then the last. I was well experienced in working with pedophiles and victims of abuse, but these families and their stories were a radical departure from anything I had ever known. Instinctively and rationally I knew that not all of these families were guilty. Who was standing up to defend the innocent ones?

My doubts about regressionism continued to mount.

Colliding Paradigms

Human thought, like God, makes the world in its own image.
ADAM CLAYTON POWELL, *KEEP THE FAITH, BABY*, 1967

I first met Dr. Pamela Freyd, the founder of the FMS Foundation, in the spring of 1993. I had invited her to come speak at the psychiatric hospital where I worked. In preparing for the meeting, there was a tremendous response from therapists, so much so that we had to relocate three times to bigger auditoriums to fit everyone in. The day finally arrived, and I met Dr. Freyd over lunch. I was impressed by the strength and intelligence of this courageous educator. Originally, she and her husband had been accused by their adult daughter, which eventually led them to assist in creating the foundation. I was keenly aware that since going public they had been the target of a great deal of hatred and rumor by the regression movement.

The auditorium was packed, and many of the regressionists I worked with were in attendance. I briefly introduced Dr. Freyd and she started her presentation. Her years in education showed. With a straightforward and quiet style she described what the FMS Foundation had discovered regarding regression trends on the national level. With well-documented evidence, Dr. Freyd drove home a very simple point: At least some portion of these recovered images were false, and we needed to better understand the phenomenon of repression and the techniques of regressionism in order to avoid false accusations and fraudulent therapies.

From the audience response, you would have thought Dr. Freyd had personally disparaged the reputation of everyone's mother in that room. Counselors starting interrupting her with angry and demeaning remarks. Others accused her of denying the reality of abuse and said that she was in fact an abuser herself. Upset and disgusted, several got up and left. Through it all I noticed that Dr. Freyd maintained an air of professionalism and caring. Her presentation had definitely touched a raw nerve in our therapeutic community. But how could professionals react in such a childish fashion? I mean, there we were, college-educated, caring healers, lashing out at someone who was simply sharing a reasonable perspective, one certainly worthy of consideration.

Welcome to the world of *paradigm shift*.

Many people assume that science proceeds in a rational, straightforward fashion. But historically, developments in science have involved a series of "revolutions," in which one way of viewing reality is violently replaced by a different one. In his seminal work, *The Structure of Scientific Revolutions*, Thomas Kuhn demonstrated that scientists have their own biases, just like the rest of us. These biases create a particular "point of view" through which they perceive and interpret problems, data, and the theories they generate.

Kuhn called this shared point of view a *paradigm*, a general framework that directs how research is conducted and the very questions that science addresses or ignores. Once accepted, a paradigm becomes a school of thought or "ism," i.e., behaviorism, evolutionism, rationalism, or, the focus of our concern, regressionism. In other words, a paradigm is like a pair of lenses through which problems are viewed and solutions developed. All of us have lenses through which we see the world, and there are certain advantages and disadvantages to every paradigm. Some "lenses" can help a person better understand a problem he has encountered, while others are inaccurate, restrictive, dangerous, and prevent a problem from being seen from other angles. I was discovering that regressionists, myself included, tended to have one lens through which they viewed their clients' problems: "Are you depressed? It's because of repressed traumas." "You're having difficulties in your marriage? It must be because of repressed traumas." Eventually everything I and other well-meaning therapists were doing was being seen through the regression lens.

Once a paradigm is established, the goal of a profession is to elaborate and confirm what the paradigm predicts, which Kuhn described as "mopping-up operations." He stated:

> Mopping-up operations are what engage most scientists throughout their careers. They constitute what I am here calling normal science. Closely examined, whether historically or in the contemporary laboratory, that enterprise seems an attempt to force nature into the preformed and relatively inflexible box that the paradigm supplies. No part of the aim of normal science is to call forth new sorts of phenomena; indeed, those that will not fit the box are often not seen at all. Nor do scientists normally aim to invent new theories, and they are often intolerant of those invented by others. Instead, normal-scientific research is directed to the articulation of those phenomena and theories that the paradigm already supplies.[15]

So the idea is to stick with what we know. But when a particular paradigm is faulty, the inconsistencies eventually begin to show. When enough contradictory evidence accumulates, the stage is set for a *paradigm shift* in which a growing number of professionals take a radical new perspective on how data, problems, and reality are interpreted. This new paradigm explains the old data in a new light and sets the stage for new explorations. But this shift isn't greeted with open arms by the old guard. Remember that entire careers, countless research projects, and numerous publications rest on the old, faulty paradigm. This process of paradigm shift that Kuhn describes is far from a neat and orderly scientific discussion. An emotional battle ensues in which the old guard rallies to protect the established system from attack by outside heretics. In a phrase, science operates on a "don't rock the boat" mentality. Those who do are viewed as troublemakers who must be silenced. Kuhn noted, "Like the choice between competing political institutions, that between competing paradigms proves to be a choice between incompatible modes of community life."[16] Because of this emotional involvement, scientists will usually do everything possible to make the established paradigm work before pondering a change. At some point, however, the older paradigm will be "overthrown" and the new one will replace it. To Kuhn the evolution of science was more of a sociological and emotional struggle than it was a rational series of steps.

Paradigms in Real Life

That's all well and good, but what's that really got to do with regressionism? Good question. Let's take a look at what paradigm shift looks like in a real-life scenario. For the last fifteen years, regression theory has played a central role in the beliefs and practices of counseling professionals. Try to imagine yourself being one of those counselors. You are convinced that there are legions of multigenerational satanists who are killing and enslaving countless victims. Thankfully you are one of the few who have been enlightened to their presence. With the leading of God and powerful techniques, you have unlocked forgotten sexual abuses and ritual tortures in several thousand clients and sounded the alarm to many more in seminars that you've conducted around the country. You're also convinced that you have survived SRA atrocities in your own childhood and are being followed by satanists, because they know you are a threat to their plans of world domination. In the intervening years you have developed a well-known reputation for delivering people from their past "chains that bind." You are a welcomed speaker as an SRA trauma expert and fellow Christians come to you for guidance. Your clients are grateful and dependent on you, and Christians around the community look up to you as a bold crusader fighting in the trenches at the very heart of the battle. Inside, there is a quiet pride that you, with just a master's degree and the Holy Spirit, have been able to be used in such a mighty fashion in the kingdom of God.

Then it happens. The facts and theories that you have been teaching are starting to be questioned. People begin to discover that your "Holy Spirit guidance" is actually a set of misleading hypnotic techniques that have simply been renamed. Your favorite authors and role models are being challenged and shown to be frauds. Increasingly, the public is becoming aware that the regressions you are doing don't hold up under scientific or biblical scrutiny. Around the country, you begin hearing that former clients are suing their regressionists and being awarded millions based on malpractice and mental-health fraud. Some of your former clients are now coming to you with questions. The pastor at your sponsoring church is also curious and wants to meet with you.

This is not simply about questioning the techniques you have been using. This paradigm shift involves your entire professional career, in fact, your entire world. Even if only a portion of your clients have had false memories, the implications are overwhelming. There's no way to know which are real and which are false. This means that thousands of recovered "memories" are suddenly open to question. With a quiet terror a thought keeps intruding, "You've perpetrated crimes against the very clients who trusted you!" With that trust, you created horrific fantasies that destroyed their lives and falsely accused families. If this were true, the crimes you have perpetrated rival the worst acts that the satanists ever did.

In the bigger picture, this is about how you view the world. There must be thousands of multigenerational satanists—the Holy Spirit would never have misled you so many times. I mean, you prayed every time for God's leading. He wouldn't give you a stone, would He? What about all those stories? And what about your own memories of ritual abuse? You've cut yourself off from all of your family, having discovered their true identity. You've hated and raged against them, publicly accused and finally forgiven them. You no longer see or hear from any of them, but that's their choice. They're the ones who choose to remain in denial. But you, you're the bold survivor committed to truth. It's impossible that what you've seen in your own recovered memories could be false. I mean, you're the expert. If anyone is going to recognize real recovered memories, you're the one!

But now some upstart band of professionals is poking around asking questions that shouldn't be asked. Thousands of parents are speaking out about their false accusations, but everyone knows that they're all perpetrators—each and every one of them. The retractors are saying they've been abused in therapy, but really they're just slipping back into denial. In a desperate effort to drown out the growing doubts, you shout even louder about, "saving the victims, the world, the Christian faith." How dare they question you. Don't they know who you are? You have years of experience, you are one of God's special agents, combating horrific conspiracies! Everyone has fallen under the deception of the satanists! They're just not brave and insightful like you! People just can't handle the truth!

But the disturbing fact is that the regressionists are the ones who can't handle the truth. The price for admitting they've been wrong, even recognizing a portion of the False Memory Crisis, is simply too much. Denial is the response they choose. Shout, quote Bible verses, cite phantom statistics and sophomoric studies, anything in an effort to drown out the growing tide of truth. But the funny thing is, truth never asks our permission, it just is. And those who fail to conform their lives to truth are ultimately doomed to be crushed by it.

Recognizing the truth of the False Memory Crisis involves a paradigm shift that is a radical departure from the world that the regressionists have created. It's not a matter of hard-core regressionists getting enough information in order to change. A person can make the choice to refuse change, no matter how much evidence is presented. As Kuhn pointed out, devotion to a paradigm is an emotional commitment, and we are endowed with the power of free will and choice. Each one of us has the power to choose life or death, truth or deception. No one can make those choices for us.

I was discovering that I had to be open to the truth, no matter what the implications were. Each moment that I was involved in regressionism I was making a choice to believe and descend ever deeper. But the good news is that this same powerful gift of free will, which had brought me into regression beliefs, could also allow me to walk out of my deception step-by-step.

I had come to understand my own deception.

Righting Wrongs

To be mistaken is a misfortune to be pitied; but to know the truth and not to conform one's actions to it is a crime which Heaven and Earth condemn.
GIUSEPPE MAZZINI, *THE DUTIES OF MAN AND OTHER ESSAYS*, 1910

What was I to do? I had been using regression techniques on my clients, and they had developed hypnotic images of abuse, right on cue. But I had come face-to-face with the reality that the regression techniques I had been taught were invalid, that they were creating delusional states of mind in my clients. Believe it or not, I was actually one of the fortunate ones. In comparison to others, my paradigm investment was minimal, and my previous years of legitimate psychological training, reasoning, and the newly uncovered facts before me were able to reach me before I slipped quietly beneath the numbing waters of regressionism.

I made one of the toughest choices of my professional career. I contacted as many of my former regression clients that I could to help them understand that their hypnotic images of trauma were not necessarily real. Some clients greeted this information with tremendous relief. I invited them to meet with me (at no charge) to hear what I had been discovering. I shared copies of studies showing the problem of False Memories, hoping to educate them. But some took great offense to my suggesting that their memories may not be real. They had come to cherish their victim role, and there was no turning back for them. My fellow regressionists were shocked that I would betray the "cause," certain that I was turning my back on victims of abuse. "Don't you believe in a real Satan?" "Your clients need you to believe them if they're to get better!" Their shock turned to rejection when they discovered that I wasn't returning to the flock. I knew that the evidence I was finding was leading me away from their firm dictates. But hard facts make for poor company. I was swimming upstream on this one, and they let me know it.

The funny thing about paradigm shift is that once your eyes have been opened to a different perspective, there's no going back to the old paradigm and pretending it's the only way to see the problem. As I came to understand the flaws and deceptions of regressionism, there simply wasn't a way for me to "unlearn," and instead I was propelled forward into the new perspectives I was discovering.

Project Middle Ground

One starts an action
Simply because one must do something.
T. S. ELIOT, *THE ELDER STATESMAN*, 1958

I had watched believers in repression completely cut themselves off from their families. In turn the accused parents were left locked out, confused, anguished, and angry. The great divide and silence that lay between the two only fed the deep wounds for both. Something had to be done. With my background as a family therapist, I was convinced that a significant part of the solution lay in opening up lines of communication. In 1993 I began an experiment that would eventually become Project Middle Ground, the first mediation program in the nation specifically designed to reach out to families torn apart by regressionism. With the permission of parents, I started contacting accusers by mail and phone. I wanted to know if any would consider a family meeting in a neutral, safe setting in which both sides could engage in dialogue about their differences. Predictably, a number of the accusers were adamant in not speaking with their parents until they confessed. But encouragingly, some were willing to meet and talk if they could be assured that they would not be told their memories were false. In turn, the parents agreed to meet if they could be assured that they would not be "ambushed" by a therapist believing they were guilty and simply in denial.

The family meetings began.

For the first time in years, family members in these meetings were able to experience safe dialogue, develop appropriate boundaries, agree to disagree, and brainstorm future options for how to increase communication. What we didn't do was engage in family therapy, i.e., figure out who was right or wrong, get the accuser to see her memories as false or the parents to confess to crimes. I was surprised by the success of the meetings and had found one of the keys I was looking for. Through Project Middle Ground, I was able to establish a nonthreatening meeting place that allowed families in conflict to have healthy communication and explore practical options for resolving their differences.

The Retractors

Gradually, my lectures and family mediation through Project Middle Ground increased. As they did I started to encounter women who were discovering that their "memories" of abuse were actually the creation of coercive counselors and recovery groups. Once they had questioned the validity of their hypnotic fantasies, these women were immediately abandoned by the regression network they had been dependent upon. As I spoke with these women, called *retractors*, I found that this was definitely new territory for me. I wanted to help but didn't know how. It was nearly impossible to even get them to talk to me. Earlier I told you how the parents had been distant, but that was nothing compared to the suspicions the retractors had about me. Here I was a psychologist and a Christian, for many retractors an exact parallel to their therapeutic abusers.

So at first, I did a lot of listening. I asked them to teach me about their experiences, which they did. Little by little these retractors began letting me into their world. I made it a point to be respectful and avoid "therapizing" them. While presenting at a seminar in Texas, I had the unique opportunity to get to know Laura Pasley, a pioneering retractor who is considered to be one of the matriarchs of the retractors nationally. She taught me volumes about retractors' experiences and because of her backing I was gradually admitted into the national retractor community, a rare and unique opportunity for any psychologist. I began to understand their experiences and feelings of anger, shame, and confusion. They were unsure of how to reconcile with their families or pull the pieces of their life back together.

The more I got to know the retractors, the more I was able to share my own thoughts and suggestions. Suddenly, more retractors were contacting me with questions they had: "How could I have seen these things so clearly?" "Am I crazy because I was able to fantasize so vividly?" "I don't know how to make it back to my family. Can you help?"

I found that my former regression beliefs and practices were a bridge into the retractors' world. I had done these therapies; I knew what retractors were talking about and how their therapists thought and worked. I was able to describe my own journey out, and I had the technical background to help educate them about the misinformation they had been taught. Usually one or more of their family members bore deep anger or hurt that their child or sibling could have made such allegations. Project Middle Ground was able to provide a forum in which the members of a family could describe their experiences, get educated about the manipulations of regression therapy, and resolve hurtful feelings toward one another. What had begun as a mediation program expanded to include restoring regression victims to wholeness and reconciling them to their families.

In 1993, Eric Nelson, a researcher in San Diego, approached me with an exciting research proposal. At that time, no studies had been published that examined the experiences of retractors on a national level, mostly because they were simply too suspicious of any "counselor types." With Laura Pasley's help, Eric and I were able to interview twenty retractors in the United States and Canada, an impressive number at the time. This led to the first national survey of retractors' experiences, which was published in a research article titled "First Glimpse." Some of the results of this study and comments by these retractors are included in the second half of this book.

What About the How?

False Memory Syndrome had given me the *what* to my questions, but it didn't provide the *how*. Regression believers and retractors both described detailed and deeply felt images of abuse. Tales of ritual torture, evil space aliens, incest, and previous lives were experienced as absolute truth. But how had they come to believe these fantasy events so strongly? This opened the door to the next step in my quest for truth. In the next three chapters we'll explore how external and internal forces can contribute to the formation of elaborate, false memories that have fed the False Memory Crisis.

Points to Remember

✓ Referred to as *decade-delayed disclosure, pseudomemories,* or *confabulations, false memory syndrome (FMS)* is the most popular name that has been given to the phenomenon in which a person experiences vivid fantasies of traumatic events which she has come to believe are real. FMS maintains a healthy balance in recognizing the tragedy of childhood abuse while also acknowledging the reality of the False Memory Crisis.

✓ Unlike the theory of repression, *false memories* are a well-established and documented phenomenon in research literature. It also stands to reason that some considerable portion of hypnotic images of incest, SRA, past lives, and space aliens is false.

✓ *Syndrome* refers to a pattern of symptoms that point toward a possible disease or condition. Professionals studying the false memory *syndrome* seek to identify the pattern that is emerging for clients who are involved in regressionism. Regression clients predictably experience severe personality change, extreme *decompensation*, high suicidal ideation, isolation from family and friends, and high dependence on therapists and group members.

✓ Abuse of children occurs in every socioeconomic class, from every walk of life. In sharp contrast, those claiming recovered traumatic memories are from a very select population (predominately white, young females, who are well-educated and in the middle- to upper-class). Accused families are middle- to upper-class, have stable marriages, and 81 percent identify themselves as active Christians.

✓ A *paradigm* is a world outlook that directs how research is conducted, problems are viewed, and solutions are developed. Paradigms are highly resistant to change and view the development of alternate perspectives as acts of betrayal.

✓ *Retractors* are survivors of regression abuse who have discovered that their hypnotic fantasies were actually false memories and the creation of coercive counselors and recovery groups.

Follow the Leader

The means prepare the end, and the end is what the means have made it.

JOHN MORLEY, *CRITICAL MISCELLANIES*, 1871–1908

Life seemed perfect, with gleaming green lawns stretching out in a Northern California valley. The Ramona family enjoyed all the benefits of an upper middle class lifestyle and a warm, close-knit family. Except Holly. Since about eighth grade, Holly had been suffering from bulimia. Finally, when she was a freshman at the University of California-Irvine, she asked her mom to find her some help. "Stevie" Ramona found a social worker named Marche Isabella, who, when initially interviewed, said that the main cause of eating disorders was child abuse, although she did wait to meet Holly before making that diagnosis. After about four months of therapy, Holly began to have "flashbacks" or memories of possible abuse, such as her dad touching her leg or tickling her. Week after week she and her therapist sifted through subtle images and random thoughts. At first, "the memories" seemed made up and unreal, but with rehearsed repetition and expansion of details, they gradually took hold. At that point, Holly was "ready" for an inpatient treatment of sodium amytal, which therapists told her was a "truth serum" (in actuality sodium amytal has been proven to confuse memories, at the same time solidifying "loyalty" to the alleged stories). The next day, she called her father and informed him that he had repeatedly raped her as a young child.

"Stevie" immediately divorced her husband. She felt a "gut reaction" that the accusations were true, although up to this point she had described her family life as "perfect." Gary also was fired from his $400,000-a-year job as a winery executive. His original disbelief turned into anger toward what he viewed as abusive quackery on the part of the counselors. The memories were "an absolute lie," obviously implanted by incompetent techniques. He filed a lawsuit against the therapists and the hospital, saying that their work with his daughter had destroyed his family. Expert witnesses from both sides of the "recovered memories" debate testified. After seven weeks of testimony, the jury awarded Gary Ramona $500,000 in damages for malpractice and damage. He

123

won in court, but that is small compensation for the loss of his children, his wife, and his career.[1]

In the previous chapters we've identified some strong clues as to how someone can develop false memories. In the next three chapters I want to elaborate a bit and help you understand how healthy, rational people can experience horrific fantasies as being real. In my experience I've found that the origins of false memories are varied. Some are external, outside of the person, while others are internally generated. In this chapter we'll examine some of the *external* contributors to false memories, which include therapist bias, media influences, hypnosis, and a subsequent condition known as brief reactive psychosis, and paranoid delusions.

I'll *See* It When I *Believe* It

People only see what they are prepared to see.
EMERSON, *JOURNALS*, 1863

One recent study found that the people most likely to see previous lives while in hypnosis were those who *believed* in past lives to begin with. Meanwhile, people who *didn't* believe in past lives were *less* likely to fantasize about past lives, even while under hypnosis. This same researcher was able to get past-life believers to vividly experience previous "lives" based on fictional stories he had written. While subjects were in hypnotic trance, he used subtle cues to direct them into visualizing his stories, and these subjects came to believe that the events they saw were spontaneous and real.[2]

In Chapter 4 we mentioned a study done on space alien abductees. Giving them a battery of psychological tests, they were not found to have greater mental disorders than the general public. However, the researchers noted that space alien abductees did have something in common—they had an active belief in space aliens *prior* to recovering memories of space aliens. It was only subsequent to this belief that they were able to experience their fantasies of abduction and experimentation by space aliens.[3]

The key point to understanding the False Memory Crisis is to know that *belief is everything*. Whether through readings or with the help of a hypnotherapist, regression believers must first have a belief system instilled in them before they can fantasize traumatic events. In science this is called the *expectancy effect*—once I *believe* it, then I'll *see* it. Notice that Christians are less prone to seeing previous lives or space alien abductions because they are not a part of our belief system. However, many Christians come to believe in multigenerational satanists and accept Freud's theory that sexual abuse can be repressed in the unconscious because these notions appeal to our worldview. Hence, while in trance, Christians are more likely to develop fantasies of ritual abuse and incest because we've already been preprogrammed to look for these traumas. As we discussed, hypnotic images of ritual abuse and forgotten incest are not necessarily more real then space alien abductions and past lives, but they are more *believable* for the Christian community. And therein lies the greatest danger: They appeal to the Christian paradigm. The Trojan Horse is dressed in Christian garb and we welcome it into the body of Christ.

So how is it that a belief system is instilled in a client? This process occurs from several sources, including a therapist's influence, popular media, and readings.

Therapists' Influence

The truth of these days is not that which really is, but what every man persuades another man to believe.
MONTAIGNE, "ON GIVING THE LIE," *ESSAYS*, 1580-1588

Before the client has even stepped into her first session, the stage is already set for traumatic fantasies because the treating regressionist has a strong belief system in place which he or she imposes upon the client. When I was doing regression therapies, I was well-indoctrinated into a complete belief system. I had attended all the right seminars, read the right books, and received the right supervision. I was prepared to find in my clients what I had been trained to find. A therapist's bias is a source of *iatrogenic influence*, a term taken from the Greek, meaning *doctor-generated* disorders. Iatrogenic influences can stem from a therapist's own history, personal agendas, poor training, or a mental disorder called *folie a deux*.

Therapist's Own History

Unresolved issues in a therapist's life can lead to a contamination in the therapeutic relationship, allowing a client to be influenced by the personal problems of his or her therapist. In psychology we refer to this process as *counter-transference*. A recent national survey has shown that 70 percent of female therapists and

33 percent of male therapists report that they have been physically or sexually abused in the past. These occurrence rates are far higher than what is found in the general population of Americans, which the studies' author acknowledges, "It's startling to me how high the rates of abuse are among the therapists we surveyed. I think this could be a motivation for some to become therapists themselves. They've been hurt emotionally and want to right that wrong by helping others."[4]

In another national study, it was discovered that therapists and pediatricians who had a history of being abused were more likely to believe allegations of abuse in their clients.[5] The implications of both of these studies are profound and set the stage for an epidemic of "false positives"—instances in which innocent people are accused of abuse crimes.

Biased Agendas

Political extremism involves two prime ingredients:
an excessively simple diagnosis of the world's ills and
a conviction that there are identifiable villains back of it all.
JOHN W. GARDNER, *NO EASY VICTORIES*, 1968

The feminist, Christian, and/or New Age social agendas of regressionists fuel a dangerous "black-and-white" view of the world, with no room for questioning in their battle to purge the world of whichever great evil they are fighting against. Part of the problem is therapists are shaped by *confirmatory bias*, in which they see evidence for their beliefs/hunches and don't allow for disconfirming evidence. It's a human frailty common to all people. It's not easy to challenge worldviews and beliefs.

A recent national study sought to determine what influences a therapist's beliefs about accusations of child abuse. The results were shocking. Of all the factors studied, the strongest was race. A therapist was more likely to assume someone is guilty of abusing a child if the accused is Caucasian.[6] Remember our findings from the last chapter, that recovered memories are almost exclusively a Caucasian phenomenon, with extremely few minorities represented. Now we start to understand one of the contributors. Therapists, well-learned in the politically correct doctrines of our times, have subtle (and not so subtle) biases, which play themselves out with deadly results. The social, political, and theological agendas that drive regressionists provide needed zeal and devotion to "the cause." Reading through regression literature one finds strong themes of sexist, anti-male rhetoric, stereotyping of all women as victims, and the concept that all males are guilty of something and need to be punished. Age-old biases and stereotypes are reworked into a scientific-sounding, therapeutic package.

Equally disturbing are the Christian regressionists' agendas. In my own practice of regressionism I turned away from a scientific and scriptural foundation, convinced that I was on a crusade for the forces of good. I truly believed multigenerational satanists were throughout the world in powerful positions, controlling international events. But because of my zeal, I was predisposed to take the next step, beyond the bounds of Scripture and into the realm of superstition and paranoia. I was acting out of strong theological and social conviction, and in turn my clients developed hypnotic fantasies that were consistent with my agendas.

This should be no surprise. We have been here before, during three hundred years of witch-hunting, during the Nazi holocaust, and during the "Red Scare" of Joseph McCarthy's era. The "true believers" have always committed the greatest evils in the name of the greatest good. Each group creates its devils to war against. The Christians of the Middle Ages blamed mythical legions of witches for bad weather, sicknesses, or cows going dry. Any traumatic event was a dark indicator that witches were afoot. And in the name of Jesus, Christians tortured, raped, and murdered hundreds of thousands of innocently accused. The crimes of the accused were never proven, but history stands in stunned silence at these atrocities of the witch-hunters. Yet, the deadly tradition of the witch-hunters continues into the present.

Poor Diagnostic Skills

Another contributor to iatrogenic contamination is poor diagnostic skills. Simply put, some of the regressionists I've met with have limited training in psychology and are not prepared to identify common disorders in their clients. Others have advanced training but ignore common disorders when making a diagnosis. There's a saying that I came across, "When the only tool you've got is a hammer, after a while everything looks like a nail." Regressionists tend to be "one-trick ponies." "Are you depressed? It must be repressed abuse. Unhappy? Repressed abuse. Addictions? Repressed abuse." You get the picture. Every problem, sin, conflict, or mental disorder is a result of repressed memories of abuse. In this world there are only victims, perpetrators, and therapeutic saviors who know which is which.

Two Christian regressionists whom I once spoke with exemplify this problem of poor diagnostic skills. Both were recognized MPD and SRA experts in their community and had large client loads. By way of formal education, they had high-school diplomas. While well intentioned, they simply did not have any foundation for understanding or treating the pathologies they stumbled across in their clients. Out of their meager training and education they were sincerely pursuing what they thought were the forces of Satan. Almost every disorder they encountered was seen as stemming from hidden abuse. With lots of "God talk" and misapplied Scriptures, they confidently declared they knew what they were doing was right because they had the leading of the "Holy Spirit" and didn't need to bother with secular training. But because of their lack of knowledge, they failed to realize that their entire therapy was based in Freudian theory and their clients' fantasies were actually a product of hypnotic techniques that had been renamed "Holy Spirit guidance."

Psychologists must adhere to an important guiding rule called the *principle of parsimony*—when two equally effective theories can explain the same phenomenon, but one explanation is simple and the other is complex, we must use the simpler explanation. A treating psychologist looks for the closest, most reasonable explanation for a disorder and begins from there, rather than relying on unusual, unproved theories. Retractors typically describe straightforward issues which they had originally entered into therapy with, i.e., depression, panic attacks, and so on. What they needed was to be correctly diagnosed and given the proper intervention. Their cases weren't that complicated. Instead their regressionists had exotic, nonscientific theories and techniques. Years later, these clients escaped from their "therapy" in far worse shape than when they went in. They still had their original issues to deal with, but now also had years of therapeutic abuse, traumatic fantasies, and destroyed relationships heaped on top.

Folie a Deux

Folie a deux is one of the most serious examples of iatrogenic influence. This is a French phrase which translates as "insanity of two." This disorder occurs when two or more people have the same mental disorder, most often a paranoid delusion with persecution themes. Typically one person dominates the relationship and is driven by a paranoid view of the world. The second person tends to be more submissive and suggestible. Their relationship is so intertwined that the dominant person's delusions transfer over to the submissive partner. The good news is that, if separated, the delusions of the submissive partner will decrease. However, the dominant partner's delusions are more entrenched and usually require extensive treatment.

You can readily see the serious complications when the treating therapist is the lead figure in *folie a deux*. A new client is hurting, looking for answers, and naive in assuming that her therapist is competent and to be trusted. In turn, the therapist offers warm, positive acceptance and speaks very confidently about repressed memory theories. Step by step, the client is pulled deeper into the delusions of the regressionist. A recent survey has noted that, of the psychologists who report having been abused as children, 40 percent had repressed "memories" that they believed to be true.[7] We have to stop and ask, "Are these psychologists really fit to provide treatment?" If they believe their own hypnotic images of abuse, are they really in a place to objectively deal with clients who make the same claims? True to Matthew 15:14, "If the blind leads the blind, both will fall into a ditch."

Through unresolved traumas, biased agendas, poor diagnostic skills, and *folie a deux*, a therapist can inadvertently harm his clients. The American Medical Association has warned:

> It is well established . . . that a trusted person such as a therapist can influence an individual's reports, which would include memories of abuse. Indeed, as the issue of repressed memories has grown, there have been reports of therapists advising patients that their symptoms are indicative—not merely suggestive—of having been abused, even when the patient denies having been abused. Other research has shown that repeated questioning may lead individuals to report events that in fact never occurred.[8]

Media Influences

All of us are influenced by the media—that's why advertising is such a major industry. Through books, articles, seminars, talk shows, and movies, many can be persuaded to buy, believe, or change to what a promoter is selling. Following Madison Avenue's lead, regression literature and popular media have played an important role in creating a belief system that people have embraced as truth.

Regression Literature

An important contributing source is the volumes of misleading regression literature that are given to clients to read. While not scientific, they contain factual-sounding theories and compelling, emotional stories. Earlier, we discussed the use of "symptoms lists," which mislead a vulnerable client into believing she has repressed memories of abuse. In our study on retractors' experiences, we discovered the seminal role that regression literature played in generating hypnotic images of trauma. Regarding *The Courage to Heal*, retractors had powerful reactions and comments. "Susan" declared: "That is a book full of suggestions, hatred, bitterness, resentment; it gives you the power to hate, fight, accuse, to rip up your own family." "Alice" stated: "[When I was twelve or thirteen] a family member told me that I had symptoms of childhood sexual abuse. She gave me *The Courage to Heal* to read. It gave me nightmares. The book said if you think you were molested then you probably were—and my family member was telling me she thought I had been molested." "Robyn" commented: "*The Courage to Heal, Secret Survivors*—I hated those books later on. When I read those books I was sick. They were very influential, very powerful, very convincing." "Carrie" agreed: "*The Courage to Heal* made me nauseous. . . . I couldn't even finish it. I was made to read *Toxic Parents*. Every time I turned around, the therapist was giving me some horrible book to read which would really upset me."[9]

Other readings have also played an important role. "Kim" stated, "I read everything. Memories were triggered by books and movies. *When Rabbit Howls* and *Suffer the Children* were passed around by group members." Alice commented, "I reprocessed the whole rape scene in the book *The Prince of Tides* as my own. Additionally, my memories of SRA came after reading *People of the Lie* by Scott Peck. We passed this book around. Women who read it got SRA memories."[10]

In all, 75 percent of the retractors reported that their delusions had been influenced by readings, including *The Courage to Heal*, *Michelle Remembers*, *Sybil*, *When Rabbit Howls*, *The Satan Seller*, *Toxic Parents*, and *Secret Survivors*. Through these readings, vulnerable clients were taught misleading theories, presented as facts, which helped indoctrinate them into the regression belief system.

Movies

In our study movies were also cited as common sources of fantasies. Fifty percent of the retractors reported developing false memories after seeing movies, including *Sybil*, *The Three Faces of Eve*, and *When Rabbit Howls*.[11] Retractors also discussed the influence of segments on *The Oprah Winfrey Show* and various videotapes. One retractor noted, "We were constantly watching videos, reading books, journaling . . . one person's memory sets up the next person's memory. Ninety percent of the memories were directly the result of videos and books."[12] Another reported that she reprocessed a scene from the movie *Deranged*, in which a deer is gutted, replacing the actors in the film with members of her family. Two other retractors, living fifteen hundred miles from each other, reported developing the same hypnotic images, which they subsequently traced to the movie *Sybil*. They reprocessed a scene in which Sybil's mother gives her a cold enema, replacing the actors with themselves and their mothers.

The Magical Powers of Hypnosis

Dreams, which, beneath the hovering shades of night,
Sport with the ever-restlessness of minds of men,
Descent not from the gods. Each busy brain
Creates its own.
THOMAS LOVE PEACOCK, *DREAMS*, 1806

Through the deadly influences of regression therapists, readings, and popular media, the client is now prepared for taking the plunge. Now that she *believes* in regressionism, she can *see* her preprogrammed fantasies through the power of hypnosis.

Everybody knows that hypnosis improves your memory. You've seen it in the movies. The killer is approaching his next victim, just as he's about do her in, he's scared off, and as the woman passes out, she catches a glimpse of his license plate. Later, she's unable recall the plate numbers. But have no fear! The hypnotist is called in to help refresh her memory. With his magical help, she is able to recall the numbers. The police race to the killer's address, just in time to arrest him and save his next victim.

Hollywood wouldn't lie to us.

Or would they?

In my investigations the misuse of hypnosis by regressionists is by far the strongest contributor to the False Memory Crisis. The notion that hypnosis and other trance-induction methods (self-induced trance, dream work, guided imagery, the use of spirit guides, etc.) are powerful tools for recovering lost memories is a popular misconception amongst therapists. Nationally, a stunning 83 percent of therapists believe that hypnosis counteracts the defense mechanism of repression, lifting repressed material into conscious awareness.[13] Sandra, the sincere regressionist we met in Chapter 2, declares, "Guided Imagery is a tool to access memory—it doesn't itself create memory."[14]

Nothing could be further from the truth. In 1985 the American Medical Association (AMA) came out with a definitive review of the research on hypnosis. The AMA concluded that hypnosis can lead to false recollections and confabulation (creating false memories), and that memories obtained through the use of hypnosis are less reliable than nonhypnotic memories. To further complicate matters, people become *more* confident about the accuracy of memories developed through hypnosis, even though they should be questioning them. The AMA stated:

> Hypnosis can also lead to increases in false recollection and confabulation. . . . There is no data to support [the theory] that hypnosis increases remembering of only accurate information. Contrary to what is generally believed by the public, recollections obtained during hypnosis not only fail to be more accurate but actually appear to be generally less reliable than nonhypnotic recall. Furthermore . . . hypnosis may increase the appearance of certitude without a concurrent increase of veracity.[15]

An experiment conducted by a psychologist at the University College in London illustrates this point. While doing a television documentary on hypnotism, Dr. Marks acquired the assistance of three secretaries at the television station. After doing a few routine experiments on hypnosis at the station office, Marks invited the three to go with him to lunch. Little did the women know that the real experiment was about to begin.

As they got out of the car at a restaurant, an "armed robbery" took place directly across the street. The three secretaries had a clear view of the entire event. They watched as the "robbers" made a noisy exit and jumped into their get-away car. Later, with the cooperation of the police and television executives, Marks hypnotized each of the women separately and questioned them about the robbery. Each was able to give a detailed recounting, including the number of perpetrators, the make and color of the get-away car, and other relevant details. The problem is that none of the three woman's stories agreed with the other. The color of the car was different for each woman, as was the number and sex of the robbers. Each retelling of the events brought out more conflicting accounts, and none of the secretaries' hypnotic images was close to accurate in describing what actually took place.[16]

Of course, the robbery was faked by Marks to show that increased accuracy in memories by using hypnosis is a farce. Remember, his experiment involved hypnosis right after the traumatic event. Imagine the amount of distortion which would occur for an event that was supposed to have happened forty or fifty years ago.

How Does Hypnosis Work?

Sleep hath its own world,
And a wide realm of wild reality,
And dreams in their development have breath,
And tears, and tortures, and the touch of Joy.
BYRON, *THE DREAM*, 1816

People react differently to hypnosis. Some people are very susceptible while others cannot be hypnotized at all. Some can even be hypnotized without their knowledge. Years ago Milton Erickson, the famous hypnotist, induced clients into a hypnotic state without their even knowing. In the same fashion, the regressionist uses words, activities, and a quiet voice to relax a person, which induces a naturally occurring state of *trance*. Once a person begins to trance, the regressionist will suggest pictures, places, scenes, and activities in order to guide the client into deeper trance and fantasy. This same process takes place in *self-hypnosis*, where a person can guide himself into his own trance state.

So what is this thing called *trance*? Trance is a common, everyday occurrence for all of us. Simply defined for our purposes, it involves an intense focus on a mental image while becoming less aware of one's physical surroundings—allowing one's mind to wander while his body is in a relaxed state. Once in trance, a person is vulnerable and responds less critically to suggestions, which is known as *hypersuggestibility*. In this state a person can be influenced to change his or her beliefs and behaviors. In addition, what one experiences seems very real and can include sight, smell, touch, relationships, and deep emotions.

Trance is what happens to you when you're driving home from work preoccupied. You look up and realize that you've driven five miles down the road without being consciously aware of driving. You glance in the rear-view mirror, wondering if you've run a red light or, heaven forbid, run somebody over. Watching a movie is another example of a natural trance state. You sit, relaxed, in a dark room where distractions have been minimized. Small, colored points of light on a large white screen form moving pictures that your mind assimilates into a whole. Actors play out dramatic performances created from fictional scripts and stories. But as we sit in a darkened room with strangers beside us, we experience a wide range of emotions: laughter, anger, fear, joy. In this natural trance state, our mind creates a vivid experience that we react to as real.

Sleeping is another example of daily, natural trance state. *Hypnagogic hallucinations* are the colorful images you see as you begin to drift off to sleep. When you're waking up, these images are referred to as *hypnopompic hallucinations*. These relaxed fantasy states and dreams contain high amounts of *daily residue*, that is, thoughts and events from the previous day. Interestingly, sleep states are one of the more common sources of recovered "memories." Fifty-eight percent of space alien abductees encounter their aliens as they are waking up in the middle of the night.[17] In a similar fashion other types of regression believers get many of their "flashbacks" during sleep states. I've had believers argue that their recovered "memories" must be real because they received them at night, with no therapist there to influence them. But the reality is the person has spent the day reading recovery literature and obsessing on horrible imaginations. That night, she lays down and her mind draws upon daily residue to create dreams. If the client had been obsessing about pink elephants, she would have dreamed about them that night. In the next therapy session, the regressionist will assert that the unconscious mind is sending repressed "memories" of abuse to the client as she sleeps. But the truth is, daily residue is reflected in the content of dream-state fantasies.

Hypnosis and Fantasy

It is important to understand that fantasy is a regular part of trance. As obvious and simple as this may seem, regressionists will disagree with this statement. Often they claim that traumatic scenes experienced in trance (hypnosis) are historically accurate and must be believed, for hypnotized clients don't make up visions of abuse. They fail to acknowledge to themselves or to inform their clients that fantasy is a large part of trance, and that even factual events can become distorted. That is why many courts don't allow hypnotically enhanced testimony; it just isn't reliable. Despite these facts, 43 percent of therapists still believe that "hypnotically obtained memories are more accurate than simply just remembering."[18]

Because fantasy and distortion are a part of trance, a process of confirmation and disconfirmation is necessary in order to find out if the images experienced by clients during hypnosis are accurate. There are no standard answers. Some patients' images may be fairly accurate, while others may involve complete fantasy. Others may be a combination of fact and fantasy. At this time there is simply no way for a therapist or client to know if a traumatic image is real without external confirming evidence. The AMA warns:

> When hypnosis is used for recall of meaningful past events, there is often new information reported. This may include accurate information as well as confabulations and pseudomemories. These pseudomemories may be the result of hypnosis transforming the subjects' prior beliefs into thoughts or fantasies that they come to accept as memories. Furthermore, since hypnotized subjects tend to be more suggestible, subjects become more vulnerable to incorporating any cues given during hypnosis into their recollections. The Panel found no evidence to indicate that there is an increase of only accurate memory during hypnosis and recognized that there is no way for either the subject or the hypnotist to distinguish between those recollections that may be accurate and those that may be pseudomemories.[19]

Research is consistent in showing basic outcomes of trance-induction techniques:

- When hypnotized a person reports increased details about an event. But there is a rise in the reporting of accurate as well as fictional information. Apart from external confirmation there is no way to tell which is which.

- Entirely fictional events that have no reference to reality can be easily created in some hypnotized subjects. These "pseudomemories" can have intricate detail and congruent emotional effect—they look and feel like a real event, both for the subject and the observer. This is particularly true for Fantasy Prone Personalities, Grade Fives, and Dissociative populations (discussed in chapter 10).

- Hypnosis produces highly suggestible states of mind in subjects. Subjects can unknowingly incorporate the immediate suggestions of the hypnotist or act on previous readings, teachings or personal expectations they had prior to being hypnotized.

- While hypnotized subjects have increased experiential fantasy in which fictional events can be experienced across all five senses.

- After hypnosis, subjects have increased levels of certitude concerning recalled information, regardless of how accurate it really is. A person can fantasize an entirely fictional event, yet post-hypnosis be very certain that it was real.

It's important to understand that hypnosis is not the problem—the misuse of hypnosis is. It is argued that hypnosis can help in reducing anxiety, phobic conditions or helping in controlling pain. There may be some validity to these claims, but this much is clear—*it is never appropriate to use trance induction techniques as memory aids without solid, external evidence to corroborate the reported information*. But I had firmly believed, and practiced, the opposite. I had regularly hypnotized clients and taken them back in time to "forgotten" traumatic events without any effort to measure their reports with objective reality. With the best of intentions, I had unknowingly deceived my clients into believing that their hypnotic images could only be true.

Brief Reactive Psychosis

"Kim," a petite brunette in her late twenties, sat in my office describing the hypnotic images she got while in regression therapy. "I could see my mom standing over the stove. She's frying a baby in a pan. She turns around and puts a fried arm on my plate.

Then she makes me eat it. I can smell the burning flesh, the taste of the arm in my mouth is nauseating." After a series of traumatic fantasies, Kim's emotional state rapidly deteriorated, and she found herself in ever-increasing amounts of therapy.

Even though her traumas were fictional, because of hypnosis Kim experienced them as real events. Subsequent to this fantasy, Kim experienced what psychologists call *brief reactive psychosis*. This is a disorder in which there is a sudden onset of psychotic symptoms, including incoherence, loose associations, delusions, inability to function, becoming a danger to one's self, and becoming dependent on others. Normally, prior to brief reactive psychosis, the level of functioning is quite good. However, when an overwhelmingly stressful event occurs, it can become too much for a person's mind to absorb, and she experiences a temporary mental breakdown. Left out of control, the person is vulnerable to the influences of those around her.

If the brief reactive psychosis is maintained beyond the period of one month, it becomes a full-blown *delusional disorder*, involving false beliefs that often include paranoid fears that someone is out to hurt her ("The satanists are out to get me." "Space aliens have been listening in on me." "My family, society, and church have conspired against me to deny the truth of my victimization."). Fantasy becomes increasingly entangled with reality. Events, past and present, are distorted in such a way as to support the person's growing paranoia. Increasingly, the person is incapacitated, leaving her more dependent on the regression leader and group members.

This is the process I saw occurring to patients while they were in the hospital. First they were told that they had all the indications of forgotten abuse; then they were given scientific-sounding books to read, and authoritative therapists and supportive group members instilled a growing belief system. Soon they were subjected to hypnosis in which they developed the expected fantasies. Their subsequent psychotic breakdowns were pointed to as evidence that they really had repressed memories—"The amount of emotion and detailed accounts in your recovered memories can only mean that these events really took place." The patient was inundated with therapists, groups, readings, and films which constantly reinforced the hideous fantasies as real. As the days turned into weeks and then months, the patient's grasp of reality continued to disintegrate and the paranoia and delusions grew. Eventually, she would cut off anyone who might challenge the reality of the fantasies and had only her "new family" to turn to for support. The very techniques which were intended to bring about healing were actually bringing about the mental destruction of the patient. In a landmark legal case, the New Hampshire Supreme Court warned:

> Therapy is recognized to be inherently suggestive. It is universally recognized that the processes involved in interactions such as psychotherapy are highly complex and undue suggestion may result. Suggestion has been found to be multi-dimensional, and may be influenced by the "hypnotizability" of the subject, the providing of misinformation, social persuasion, and interrogation. . . . Use of so-called guided imagery, a process by which a therapist directs a client's visualization, is considered highly suggestive. Age regression therapy, by which a patient is encouraged to return to an appropriate time in his or her childhood and to experience an event as that child would, is considered suggestive. Furthermore, a therapy by which a therapist communicates to his or her client a belief or confirmation of the client's beliefs or memories can be highly suggestive. . . . It is inappropriately suggestive for a therapist to communicate to a client his or her belief that a dream or a flashback is a representation of a real life event, that a physical pain is a "body memory" of sexual abuse, or even that a particular memory recovered by a client is in fact a real event.[20]

Now we begin to understand how someone quite healthy can create violent fantasies they come to believe as real. First, through a therapist's influence, "symptoms" lists, and regression literature a client develops a belief system. These influences can contribute to daily residue, which finds its way into her dream state. These dreams, in turn, are used as confirmations of what the regressionist has implanted in the client. With these stages, the expectancy effect is put into place. The client believes that there is something hidden within her. Through the subsequent use of hypnosis, she can begin to look for fantasy images that comply with her expectancy effect. Finally, this can lead to a brief reactive psychosis in which the shock of violent fantasies overwhelms her and leads to psychotic behaviors and greater dependency. If the pressure is maintained it will eventually lead to a full-blown paranoid delusional disorder.

Points to Remember

✓ The key point to understanding the False Memory Crisis is to know that *belief is everything*. Whether through readings or with the help of a therapist, regression believers must first have a belief system instilled in them before they can fantasize traumatic events.

✓ *Iatrogenic influences* can stem from a therapist's own history, personal agendas, poor training, or *folie a deux* and can have a seriously adverse effect on clients.

✓ Once a client is indoctrinated into a regression belief system, she can then see her preprogrammed fantasies through the power of therapist- or self-induced hypnosis. Various hypnotic techniques create a naturally occurring state of *trance* in which a client experiences fantasy images as if they were real.

✓ Once in trance, a person is vulnerable and responds less critically to suggestions. This is known as *hypersuggestibility*, in which a person can be influenced to change her beliefs and behaviors.

✓ Research is consistent in showing that trance-induction techniques create highly suggestible and delusional states in which clients have: 1) decreased ability to accurately recall historical events, 2) increased experiential fantasy, and 3) increased levels of certitude concerning the accuracy of recall (even though the images are actually less reliable).

✓ Once a client is inducted into regression belief and subjected to hypnosis, she is vulnerable to *brief reactive psychosis* which can lead to long-term *paranoid delusions*. In this state she becomes increasingly psychotic and vulnerable to the influences of those around her.

Join the Club

We are so fond of one another, because our ailments are the same.
JONATHAN SWIFT, *JOURNAL TO STELLA*, 1711

"Elizabeth" sits in my office, dazed and angry. She's only recently come out of regressionism and is trying to make sense out of what has happened to her. She is very bright. With a doctorate in science, she works on extremely technical and highly classified government projects. She has an intellect that surpasses those of most clients I've worked with. But that only makes it worse. "With all my intelligence, I can't believe that I fell into this. I'm ashamed that I let them do this. I just don't understand how it happened!"

It began with going to a therapist for problems with depression and alcohol abuse. This led to a series of inpatient treatment programs. She explained: "Last year my humanity was shredded by psychoanalytic vultures. Barely touching the fringes of the events that transpired sucks me back into the fear and pain. My voice rises, my speech becomes quicker, my thoughts race. Through therapy I was led to believe that if I could make my memories as continuous as possible from my first memories to my present age, I could then understand my current behavior. Therapists explained that many of my memories were repressed when I was a child because they were too traumatic and overwhelming. Recently they were resurfacing through nightmares, panic attacks, and flashbacks because it was only now that my psyche was able to handle the traumas. I was assured that if I could recover the repressed memories during therapy and deal with them, I would be able to find the underlying reason for my suicidal drinking. What they told me sounded right, and I was desperate to find a reason for my depression. The therapists I put my faith and trust in were trained professionals from well-known institutions. When I asked them questions, I believed what they told me—I knew that I didn't have the answers. What they described sounded logical and I was willing to give it a try. But given the condition I was in, I wasn't really capable of making good decisions. I placed my complete faith and trust in these professionals.

"To state it concisely, I was mind-raped and soul-raped in the name of repressed memory theory. I believe tampering with people's memories is absolutely reprehensible. I was misdiagnosed with post-traumatic stress disorder. I was given improper medications and analysis that almost cost me my life on many occasions. After each treatment center I would come back in just as bad or worse shape than I left. If I ever hear the following from anyone else in this world I will vomit: 'I must go through the pain to reach the other side.' Yeah, right! I think it should be set to elevator music.

"The memory work was a never-ending, lifelong process. I was uncovering the 'truth' through dreams, recurring nightmares, imagery, visualization techniques, anger work, peer-pressure, and more. By the time I got to my final inpatient treatment center I believed I was going to have to deal with my flashbacks and panic attacks for a long time, so I was learning how to ground myself. I was having nightmares, which were getting worse the more therapy I had. This much was clear to me: I wasn't getting better.

"I began to ask questions. There was always some prophetic, profound, deep jargon sort of an answer to any and to all questions I asked. It was a pat answer with no meaning. I remember some unanswered questions I asked. 'If the traumatic events hurt so badly when they happened, why do I have to go through them again as an adult? How come I have only bad memories and no good ones? What happened to the good?' I remember walking around a whole day trying to remember anything even sort of good, such as holidays. They always started out as good but ended bad. I had no more good memories. Once again, I received pat, therapeutic windbag answers, more beating around the bush. No direct answers.

"Day by day, the core of who I was, my memories, my beliefs, my feelings were altered to coincide with false realities and atrocities that became utter truth to me. My physical body was there; my feelings and emotions were like nerves in the roots of teeth exposed to air—painful, excruciating. I shudder and feel physically nauseous when I think of the enormity of the repressed memory therapy I and many others were subjected to at [an inpatient mental health facility]. Through the events last year I learned how to survive terror tactics such as restraints, quiet rooms, suicide watches, and drugs used when anyone became angry. I've never seen so many hurt so badly in places they went to be healed, yet day by day never getting any better."

Toxic Groups

Do not be misled: "Bad company corrupts good character."
THE APOSTLE PAUL, 1 CORINTHIANS 15:33, (NIV)

Elizabeth's story is repeated in thousands of lives across the nation. A key element in her induction was the role that group members played in encouraging and feeding memory recovery. My work with retractors through Project Middle Ground revealed the powerful influences that their recovery groups had on them. In our study 93 percent of retractors who developed fantasies in group therapy reported that similar or identical memories had been described by other members.[1] "Sally" noted:

> When other participants described emotional and graphic scenes, the emotional degree influenced me more. Details influenced me more. . . . I used to encourage the other women to describe graphic scenes so that it might "trigger" my memories. I thought the only way to feel better was to force the memories out of me. After hypnosis the memories got more detailed and bizarre. We had to work at it to keep the memories coming, otherwise we would slip into "denial" and begin doubting. It took lots of work. We talked about denial a lot.[2]

"Allison" agreed. "If you don't have a memory you feel like you have to come up with one to compete with everybody."[3] "Susan" added, "We had very similar alters and memories. One woman would feel left out because she didn't have a particular alter everyone else had, and she wanted it."[4]

In my pursuit to better understand the formation of false memories, my studies and interviews helped me to appreciate how toxic group dynamics can help pull healthy, intelligent people into fearful and zealous beliefs. You see, all of us have various groups we identify with—churches, professional organizations, civic clubs. Groups provide an important social linking that helps us in a variety of ways. But not all groups are beneficial; some groups are actually unhealthy and have a detrimental effect. We've attached different labels in describing these, including "gangs," "hate-groups," "religious/therapeutic cults," and so on. I prefer to use the term *toxic groups.*

Groups exert overt and subtle pressures that create conformity in their members. *Conformity* can serve positive purposes, creating an important social force for a society to maintain moral conduct in its citizens. But group conformity can also have a negative influence, persuading individuals to violate their own principles and even deny objective reality. A person's desire and need to conform can actually be used against him in a destructive way. Two classic studies shed light on this process. One researcher did a study in 1935 in which people altered their perceptions of reality in order to fit with their group's consensus. He used an optical illusion, called the *autokinetic effect,* in which a pinpoint of light shown in a darkened room appears to move, but actually the point of light remains perfectly still. First, a subject was placed in a darkened room alone, and he or she described the point of light as moving in a variety of directions (a normal response). Next, a group of subjects was placed in the same darkened room to repeat the task. This time, because of natural group processes, all the subjects became united in seeing the light moving in one specific direction. Finally, each subject was again put into the darkened room alone. Guess what. This final time individuals reported that the light was moving in a specific direction, the same one that their group had decided on earlier. Remember, the light never was moving in the first place. But the group's influence held its effect on each person's perception, even after the group was gone from the room.[5]

A similar study was done in 1956. A researcher had groups of subjects perform a very simple visual discrimination task. They were shown three vertical lines on a card and asked to point to the one that was closest in length to a separate comparison line. What the real subjects didn't know was that their other group "members" were actually researchers who were part of the experiment. It was prearranged that these "fakes" would pick a clearly *incorrect* line. The real subject was asked to point to the correct line while the fake members pointed unanimously to a wrong one. You guessed it, only 25 percent of the time was the subject able to remain completely independent and not give in to the misleading opinions of the majority.[6]

Group conformity is a natural process. We conform for two basic reasons. One is that other people in our lives provide a social reference point that helps us gauge acceptable conduct, what is important, the nature of reality. Another reason is because it's natural to avoid rejection and desire to be approved of by others. Conflicting perceptions create a state of *cognitive dissonance* in which we experience a great deal of internal discomfort because what we feel is in contradiction with people around us. Are they right or are we? Which way do we go? What if we make the wrong decision? We don't want to be rejected, the odd person in the crowd. People will go to great lengths, even sacrificing health and reality, in order to quiet the dissonance they feel within them.

It's no mistake that recovery groups are a weekly part of a regression believer's diet. Studies have shown that group discussion intensifies the opinions of like-minded people—individuals hear additional arguments for their own viewpoints and discover that others are more supportive when they express support of the group consensus. The group's agenda is promoted away from any kind of questioning or individual dissent. The new convert begins to vocalize her new perceptions in a stronger fashion the longer she stays. Interestingly, people who have higher self-esteems are actually less likely to conform to inappropriate group pressures. But notice that people with high self-esteem aren't very likely to be in therapy in the first place; those with low self-esteem are.

Groupthink

All groups are subject to a process called *groupthink*, a phenomenon in which a group's desire for harmony and approval leads to the loss of critical judgment. Symptoms of groupthink include a sense of invulnerability ("we could never be wrong"), an unquestioned belief in their own moral superiority, pressure on dissenters to conform, an illusion of unanimity, collective rationalizations, a stereotyping of out-groups, the institution of politically correct thoughts, and individual self-censorship. The conditions which breed groupthink include high cohesiveness, isolation from outside contact, and a directive leader.

If you're honest with yourself, you'll see that groupthink is something we've all experienced in varying degrees, regardless of our group's political or theological persuasions. Sociologists' concerns begin when this process becomes more extreme and a group is increasingly isolated from differing perspectives, when it loses its ability to doubt itself and to ask questions. Here are some "red flags" to watch out for:

Unquestioned Leadership

The leader typically is a respected person who is seen as having special powers of discernment or insight and is never to be contradicted by his or her followers.

Special Knowledge

A group believes it has secret knowledge or privileged status of which the rest of the world has been deprived. People can only become enlightened by joining its circle and thereby obtaining these "truths."

Altered States of Consciousness

A definite red flag is the use of altered states of mind to obtain hidden "truths." Toxic groups downplay the use of reasoning and normal skills of perception and instead promote various transcendental states as pathways to truth.

Manipulation/Deception

Watch out for a group that uses deceptive techniques in attracting new members and keeping them within their ranks. Later in this chapter we'll explore some common techniques, including *double-binding, paralogical thinking,* and *fear tactics.*

High Dependency/Lack of Autonomy

Toxic groups demand absolute dependency and allegiance from members. Any family or friends who question the member's new "truths" are "heretics," "unbelievers," or "in denial" and must be excommunicated until they come to see the "light." This results in the new member bonding with his or her newfound family and away from old family and friends. Autonomous thinking is discouraged or forbidden, with the will of the group becoming the member's first priority.

Paranoia

Another red flag is an "us against them" mentality. Competing groups or outsiders are viewed as desiring to harm the group members and various "devils" are created to explain away critics. Devils can include family members, friends, legal institutions, and churches who dare to question the group's truths.

The Question of Cults

What exactly constitutes a cult? Definitions differ. A *theological perspective* focuses on a group's *teachings*, as in a group which claims to be part of a recognized religion, but its actual teaching represents a serious departure from orthodox tenets. For example, if a particular group claimed to be Christian but taught that Christ was only one of many messiahs, this would be defined as a cult since its teaching represents a serious departure from traditional Christianity. In contrast, a *sociological definition* of a cult emphasizes the dynamics which occur within a group, with less of an emphasis on its teaching.

As we continue I want to offer a precaution: Just because you or I disagree with a particular group's teachings doesn't mean the group is "destructive," "unhealthy," or a "cult." The question of a group's harmful nature is not an "either/or" question, and it is not my intention to label all regression groups as cultic. Certainly some of them are, but my concern is broader than the label cult implies. Imagine a spectrum line: On one end lie healthy group dynamics and on the other are toxic characteristics. We determine the level of harm a group can do based on where it falls on the spectrum line. Regression groups represent a dangerous closed system that prevents members from hearing differing perspectives or questioning the group doctrine. They include dangerous levels of all the characteristics we've just discussed. The question we face is not, "Is regressionism a cult?" Instead we must ask a broader question: "To what degree do regression groups reflect the toxic dynamics described in this chapter?"

Ideal Candidates for Toxic Groups

Bob Fellows travels throughout the country teaching college groups the different kinds of manipulations and deception methods that are used by harmful groups. In his book, *Easily Fooled*, he lists common characteristics of people who are most vulnerable to cultic influences. He emphasizes that anyone can be fooled, but especially people who

- Are under stress
- Are in a transition in their lives
- Have a tendency toward dependency

- Are unassertive
- Are gullible
- Want simple answers to complex questions
- Are idealistic
- Are disillusioned with the world or their culture
- Are naive
- Have an unfulfilled desire for spiritual meaning
- Are attracted to trance-like states of mind
- Are unaware of how groups can manipulate people
- Have recently had a traumatic experience
- Do not know how the mind and body affect each other
- Lack skills in critical thinking and logic
- Lack knowledge of methods of deception.[7]

As you take a look at this above list, consider some of the common reasons someone goes into therapy. *Under stress, in transition, dissatisfied, traumatized, desperate for answers to distress*—the client is off-balance, seeking help, and paying good money for the answers the regressionist provides. With openness and trust, she sets aside critical thinking and is left vulnerable to scientific-sounding theories and misapplied hypnotherapy. Ironically, the therapist's office, which is designed as a place for healing, is the ideal setting for being inducted into a toxic group.

Target populations for recruitment into toxic groups are people between the ages of eighteen to twenty-eight, a critical time of life in which people are experiencing life transitions, stresses, personal uncertainty, loneliness, and disappointments. Contrary to popular belief, recruits into religious and therapeutic cults are typically "normal" people. They are simply disenchanted with life, and frustrated with school or career pursuits. They are bored and unhappy. In this mode they set out to find the reason for their unhappiness. For a price, the leader and group are there to supply the answers.

Remember the finding in Chapter 8 that recovered memories occur for predominantly white, educated, middle- to upper-middle-class clients? One of the things we've discovered about religious and therapeutic cults is that they target more highly educated populations that tend to come from middle- to upper-middle-class families. Few racial or ethnic minorities are recruited. There's a practical aspect to targeting this segment of the population—money. Simply put, this is the population with the best insurance. A clinical psychologist explains what he discovered as he reviewed mental-health claims for insurance companies. Beginning in the late 1980s, he noticed a startling pattern in the claims involving MPD patients: Most of them had generous insurance policies.

> The focus was generally on patients with very rich benefits plans and I would find, in some cases, that large numbers of people from single employers with those types of plans would suddenly be presenting with this diagnosis an incidence of multiple personality way beyond anything reasonable that could be expected for a given population of individuals. So there was a targeting of the richer benefits plans. [In investigating these claims] I was met with the most hostile responses that I came across in all the years I'd done any kind of case management or clinical supervision, beginning with discounting the credibility of myself and the board-certified, experienced psychiatrists and psychologists that I used, extending on to rather strange suggestions, at times, that I might be somehow related to these satanic cults or the organizations I worked for.[8]

It's tempting to think that people who get involved with toxic groups are "asking for it" and are somehow defective. But generally people don't go looking to join a cult. They get recruited while looking for something to better their lives. This hunger for peace and fulfillment leaves them open to the false promises of a toxic group. It's our belief in our own invulnerability that opens us to a group's influence. The reality is that it can happen to anyone, given the right timing and circumstances.

Steps for Induction into Toxic Groups

We've discussed common characteristics of toxic groups and their potential recruits. But how is the new recruit actually inducted? It's clear that a person doesn't wake up one day and suddenly decide to abandon her life, family, finances, health, and identity and join a harmful group. Induction incorporates a step-by-step process by which a recruit is gradually brought into the fold. Steve Hassan has written a best-seller, *Combatting Cult Mind Control*. His writings offer valuable insights into how cult dynamics function. He describes three essential stages: *Unfreezing, Changing,* and *Refreezing*.[9]

Unfreezing

Controlled Environment: A key ingredient for induction involves controlling a new recruit's environment. This control allows misinformation, group pressures, and authoritative pronouncements to erode the recruit's critical judgment. She will naturally begin to doubt herself and defer to the reality the group and "experts" are presenting. This was the disturbing process I had watched patients go through. As I was working at the psychiatric hospital, new patients, disoriented and desperate for answers, were brought into a completely controlled environment. Typically any contact with outside family members or friends was forbidden as a part of establishing a "therapeutic milieu." In this completely controlled, locked-down environment, the patient was continuously indoctrinated day and night through numerous modalities into regression dogma by trauma "experts," group sessions, and readings. Any influence away from regressionism was completely removed, and the patient had to buy the party line if she was to "get better" and be allowed to leave. And to top it off, hospitals were paid massive amounts of money from insurance companies for providing the indoctrination. A cult could never create a better setup than the psychiatric hospital.

Unconditional, positive regard: "People can be induced to swallow anything, provided it is sufficiently seasoned with praise," wrote Molière. He was right. For the recruit, the actual propaganda of the toxic group is secondary to the fundamental needs it meets in her life. My experience has shown that the process of recovered memories is a mutual venture; the new recruit initially chooses to embrace the paradigm that the regressionist offers. They experience a tremendous amount of *secondary gain,* which is the reinforcement or "payoff" that one can receive for taking on the role of victim. By choosing the regressionist's reality, the recruit receives gratifying support and affirmation from her respected leader and group members. Cult experts refer to this technique as *"love bombing."* The group provides acceptance, community, fellowship, a sense of belonging, black-and-white answers, safety—needs we all have. But the ability to choose is only in the beginning. The deeper the recruit gets into memory recovery, the more she becomes controlled. The recruit's freedom of thought is gradually exchanged for all the positives the toxic group offers.

Radical new worldview: In the Unfreezing stage, the recruit is taught a new worldview—discarding former ways of thinking and perceiving. This leaves her natural defenses and lines of reasoning disarmed while she's indoctrinated into the group's worldview. The regression client discovers that, rather than having grown up in a normal family, she was actually the victim of years of satanic abuse, sexual assault, repeated space alien visitations, and/or prior lives. The "old" methods of remembering and perceiving reality are replaced with new ones. The past is rewritten in such a way as to distort longtime relationships into something evil, and those in the present are either "one of us" or "one of them." For the new recruit the world takes on a black-and-white quality, filled with victims, perpetrators, and those who are in denial. Hassan states:

> The recruits are told how bad the world is and that the unenlightened have no idea how to fix it. This is because ordinary people lack the new "understanding" that has been brought by the leader. The leader is the only hope of lasting happiness. Recruits are told, "your 'old' self is what's keeping you from fully experiencing the 'new truth.' Your 'old concepts' are what drag you down. Your 'rational' mind is holding you back from fantastic progress. Surrender. Let go. Have faith."[10]

Alternate states of consciousness: Trance-states are promoted in cults as the great highway to hidden secrets. Normal powers of reasoning or remembering are actually a distraction from healing. Whether through hypnosis, trance-writing, "spirit guides," or higher states of consciousness, the new convert is promised access to hidden realms.

Manipulation and deception: Regression groups rely on psychobabble, fraudulent "symptoms" lists, pseudoscientific theories, misuse of Scriptures, suggestible states of mind, isolation, and group coercion to induct new members. The new client is never informed that hypnotic techniques have been shown to lessen accurate recall, lead to suggestible states of mind, and create exotic fantasies that can be experienced as real. They aren't told that repression is a controversial theory or informed that the journey they are about to embark upon will lead to never-ending therapies, tens or hundreds of thousands of dollars in bills and hospital stays, complete termination from their family of origin and lifelong friends, severe personality change, suicide attempts, divorce, loss of job, and destroyed personal functioning. The recruit only discovers these price tags as she is drawn deeper into the fold.

Paralogical thinking: The most effective cult doctrines are those which are unverifiable. Paralogical thinking involves a false reasoning in which an individual or group distorts reality in order to make information consistent with their worldview. Regular examples of paralogical thinking that I encounter with regression believers include:

- "All pedophiles seek to be well thought of, my father is well thought of, therefore my father must be a pedophile."

- "A client can't use ordinary memory processes because they don't apply to traumatic events."

- "We can't prove the *theory* of repression because the *process* of repression can't be studied."

- "All the evidence proving a repressed memory from decades [or centuries] ago has been covered up by the perpetrators [satanists, space aliens, secret government forces]."

- "Lack of evidence is actually proof that the abuses took place."

- "The perpetrator's lack of memory of abusing his daughter is evidence that he has pushed his criminal acts out of conscious awareness. No memory is even more evidence that he committed the crime."

Under closer examination paralogical thinking is actually nonsensical. But for the new recruit it creates a confusing state in which trusted authorities are saying things that, on the surface, sound almost logical.

Double binds: This is a tremendously effective technique in regressionism. It involves forcing a person to do what the toxic leader wants, but at the same time gives an illusion of choice. "You came to therapy because things are not working out in your life, because you're dysfunctional. By not committing yourself to therapy, you continue to be dysfunctional, which is even more reason that you need to be doing regression work. You want to get better, don't you? If you knew how to do that yourself, you wouldn't have come here for treatment. Your faulty thinking is what brought you here in the first place." Like paralogical thinking, the double bind is completely disorienting for the recruit, actually leaving her guilty for having doubts about therapy. Even her doubts are turned around to show her that she needs to be in regressionism.

Stereotyping:

"Prejudice is the conjurer of imaginary wrongs, strangling truth, overpowering reason, making strong men weak, and weak men weaker."
                                                    JOHN MACDUFF

With this technique, anyone outside of the group is no longer dealt with as an individual, but as a stereotyped class. Loaded language is used as a subtle reinforcement of toxic group indoctrination, i.e., those who question the group's teachings are "in denial of the truth," "infidels," "the establishment." Recovery groups will always refer to a member's parents as "perpetrators" or "abusers" instead of "the accused" or "suspects." Rather than talking about her father or her mother in specific, real terms, the recruit learns to describe her parent as one of "them." "Of course your parents denied abusing you—satanists always deny abusing children." The recruit no longer addresses her parents but rages against an entire world filled with perpetrators. These sweeping generalizations produce a negative perception, called *prejudice*, which is highly resistant to allowing any contradictory information. When someone's parent has been described as a perpetrator, for the client there is no evidence allowed in that would disconfirm that conclusion. In my dealings with regression believers I'll often ask a basic question: "If someone were innocent, what would be the signs—how would you know?" The regression believer is typically dumbfounded. She's had extensive training in reading signs of guilt, but she's never considered how to tell when someone is innocent.

Changing
After the Unfreezing stage is completed, the recruit is now ready for "Changing." Hassan describes the stage of Changing as involving the acquisition of a new identity—new behaviors,

thoughts, and emotions—that fill the void left by the disintegration of the old self. Many techniques used in the Unfreezing phase are continued in the Changing stage.

Preventing dissent: "Sally," a retractor in our study, commented, "About half of the women in the group stated . . . 'I have been sexually abused by my father, but I don't have my memories yet. . . .' This reinforces—it is 'majority rules,' so 'many people are buying into it, how can it be wrong? I have to go with it.'"[11] "Margaret," a retractor as well, reported: "The therapist would say, 'This is a situation which probably occurred. Now relax and tell us how it happened. . . .' The group peer pressure was directed at the person to remember the abuse."[12] Conflicting views and questions are forbidden in regression groups. The notion that even some of the repressed images are fantasies is not tolerated. To allow for that possibility is to allow for the questioning of all hypnotic images. Compliance is typically accomplished through an appeal to the new convert's group loyalty. "If you question your own recovered memories, that means you're also questioning the memories of others in the group. That would be perpetrating further violence against them. You wouldn't want to do that, would you?"

Social and psychological dependence: These are promoted and independent decision-making is minimized. For example, regression believers usually allow their therapists to filter their mail, making decisions on what letters they can or cannot receive. The clients are told that they are simply not strong enough to make their own decisions, and that they have to give themselves completely over to the care of the therapists and groups.

Refreezing

Once a recruit has been taken through the stages of Unfreezing and Changing, she is now ready to move into the final stage of "Refreezing"—to be created a "new woman," with a new family, identity, reality—and a blinding fear to keep her in line.

Commitment and conforming building processes: Commitment-building processes play an important role in binding the individual to a toxic group and generating unquestioning devotion. It is essential that the member now denigrate her former, unenlightened self. During Refreezing the client's memory of her former life becomes increasingly distorted. Memories of positive events are forgotten or reshaped into dark revisions and the focus is kept on negative events (real or fictional). Recurrent themes of sacrifice and renunciation are designed to reinforce new beliefs. True believers must be willing to sacrifice all of their former lives, particularly any illusion of a caring family, in order to obtain true psychological wholeness. The toxic group comes to form the member's true family, and some cults will even have the member take on a new name. This is an essential step for maintaining dependency in members. By destroying any bridges leading away from the group, the member becomes trapped and has nowhere to turn as the cost of staying becomes more severe.

Regressionists often recommend that their clients "divorce" their parents and even change names. The regression manual *The Courage to Heal*, instructs readers to change their names in order to establish their own definition of themselves. The authors give an example of a woman, Rachel Bat Or, who gathered her friends in a name-changing ceremony. She invited nine friends to form a *minyan* (in Jewish tradition, a *minyan* is the minimum number of men required to hold religious services). After casting a circle, they invited the spirits of the south, east, west, and north to join them in their ceremony. Then Rachel read poems about herself, while the circle of nine listened. After they were finished discussing their names, Rachel had her friends write down her old name on a piece of paper and throw it into a moving body of water.[13]

"No passion so effectively robs the mind of all its powers of acting and reasoning as fear."
EDMUND BURKE, *A PHILOSOPHICAL INQUIRY INTO THE ORIGIN OF OUR IDEAS OF THE SUBLIME AND BEAUTIFUL*, 1756

Threats:
During the recruit's induction into the toxic group, he or she is initially drawn in by attractive offerings: acceptance, sure answers, a sense of privilege. But once in, the novelty wears off and the promises of healing begin to fade. In place of the promises, the member begins to experience an escalating price tag for continued involvement. The "love bombing" is gradually replaced by fear, guilt, and shame to keep the member "in line."

As the group member loses the original motivation that brought her into the fold, the toxic group must now make use of fear as the primary reason for staying. Research has shown that group members join closer together when they are taught that lack of loyalty will hurt the group or when they perceive hostility from an outside enemy. Accordingly, regression groups utilize two sources of fear in keeping members "in check"—internal threats and external threats. Regression therapists use *threats from within* to reinforce; they threaten clients with sanctions should they ever consider questioning or leaving the group. Failure to get better (the initial promise of the regressionists) is now shown to be the member's fault—she simply isn't trying hard enough, she's still in denial, she doesn't want to get better. This way, regression therapy isn't to blame for failing to heal, the member is. This leads to a double bind—the fact that you're not getting better means that you have to apply yourself to regression therapy even more. Group members come to believe that they could never be happy or fulfilled outside of the recovery group, that their journey to psychological wholeness and self-actualization would be derailed. They simply can't picture themselves as being happy away from the group.

The internal threats take on an increasingly aggressive form. Retractors have revealed that their therapists threatened to hurt them and their families if they decided to leave the group. For example, a regressionist might threaten to contact Child Protective Services to report that the retractor was abusing her children. This follows the reasoning that if the client goes back into "denial," she is bound to repeat the victimization against her own children.

"Margaret," a retractor, stated, "I had a threat from my therapist that if I questioned my memories, if I went 'into denial,' then I would be sent to a state hospital and I wouldn't get better."[14]

"Susan" noted, "I constantly questioned them [the memories]— that's when the medicine was changed. If you take enough drugs you can remember about anything. Also, the therapist would threaten to send me to a mental hospital, and tell me that I would lose custody of my child, if I didn't confront my family and accuse them based upon my memories."[15]

"Nancy" said, "I always felt pressure from the therapist, she just kept pushing me and pushing me. I always knew my brother had sexually abused me, but she kept pushing me to think that it was my father, because everyone else in the group had been abused by their fathers, [and] I was pressured into coming up with something."[16]

"Martha" commented, "I was in the hospital with a therapist in a quiet room. He was trying to hypnotize me for the third time, in an attempt to get memories. He became angry because I couldn't get memories, he said I didn't want to. He gave me 10 minutes to get a memory. I became scared, and I made up a memory to make him happy. It wasn't right—it didn't feel right."[17]

"Kathy" noted that she was hospitalized by her therapist because she wouldn't develop satanic ritual abuse memories like everyone else in her survivor group. "I didn't have SRA memories. The therapists put me in the hospital for 8 weeks until I remembered SRA. [Finally] I mimicked SRA flashbacks because I had seen them a hundred times in group. I did this to get out. I was out in one week, and I never went back [to that group]. I rejected the SRA memories immediately upon release."[18]

"Betty" states, "The more I expressed that they weren't real, that I was lying and making them up, they told me that was my denial coming up to protect me, I needed to believe the memories . . . I told my therapist that this was all false therapy, then she put me in the hospital. That was the worst thing of all, having the courage to say that this isn't true, that is when they really bombard you."[19] "Rachel" adds, "They kept pressing me—they would say you don't love your kids, you are in denial, you have abused the children, you are going to lose your husband and your children."[20]

In addition to internal threats, members are taught that an attempt to leave the safety of the group invites physical harm from outside. Hassan explains, "In every destructive cult I have encountered, fear is a major motivator. Each group has its devil lurking around the corner waiting for members to tempt and seduce, to kill or to drive insane. The more vivid and tangible a devil the group can conjure up, the more intense is the cohesiveness it fosters."[21] The "devil" for the feminists is the evil of white, Christian men. For the Christian regressionist, it is the evil of multigenerational satanists who create the calamities of the world. The devil for the New Agers is the repressive Western Christian culture which denies the reality of past lives. Space alien believers fight against a close-minded government which has covered up the truth. What each of them share is a certainty that the "evil ones" will destroy them if they ever leave the safety of the group.

Points to Remember

✓ Toxic groups create conformity, cognitive dissonance, and levels of "groupthink" which can seriously alter an individual's perception of reality. The common characteristics of people seeking therapy make them ideal for induction into toxic-group dynamics.

✓ The first stage for induction into toxic groups is referred to as *Unfreezing* and includes a controlling environment, unconditional positive regard, a radical new worldview, promotion of alternate states of consciousness, manipulation and deception, paralogical thinking, double-binding, and stereotyping of "outsiders."

✓ The second stage is *Changing* and includes preventing dissent in members and creating social and psychological dependence.

✓ The final stage is *Refreezing* and includes commitment and conforming building processes and the use of internal and external threats.

10

Monsters from Within

Let us not seek our disease out of ourselves; 'tis in us, and planted in our bowels; and the mere fact that we do not perceive ourselves to be sick, renders us more hard to be cured.

SENECA, *CONTROVERSIAE*, 1ST CENTURY

For as long as she could remember, Diana's mind was filled with dark shadows and action-packed battles with assailants and disasters. As a girl, she would drift off during classroom lectures, spinning wildly vivid and detailed adventures with herself shining in triumph. "I always thought about things that tended to be out of the normal experiences. They didn't feel like they were the usual little daydreams. They were different—more real."[1] And for Diana, they had a detailed and intense feel to them.

As an adult, Diana became interested in spiritual warfare. Eagerly reading popular books and attending seminars and group meetings on the subject, she came to believe that there were powerful satanic forces behind global events. After experiencing bouts of depression, she thought that perhaps her mind was trying to make her aware of past secrets. When a childhood friend called to tell her that she and Diana had watched their fathers brutally kill adults and children in satanic rituals, it seemed to make some sense. "As she was talking, these images came into my mind. It seemed so detailed, so real. It was like watching a movie."[2] She sought out a Christian therapist who was experienced in recovering lost memories, and the nightmare began. After seeing her Christian regressionist for individual session work, Diana went to an inpatient program that specialized in treating victims of satanic ritual abuse. There Diana was able to "recall" further crimes, including a time that she crushed a man's skull in a ritualistic fashion, heaving a rock that was far too immense for her to lift. The therapists probed for more stories. If nothing came to mind, "They would say, 'Oh, we didn't do too well today.'"[3] She explained, "I wanted to please them, and get to the truth."[4]

Most powerful of all were the group sessions, where one was accused of hurting the whole group if horrible details were withheld or questioned. "They were real adamant in their belief that any image that came to my mind had to be true. If you say, 'This image of abuse is just a fantasy,' it's a threat to the whole group. If you don't believe your own memories, how can you believe theirs?"[5] Any doubts that she expressed further proved the accusations, as this was the expected "denial" that all victims felt.

These memories eventually led her to cooperate with the local police, who were zealously investigating the allegations of murders and abuse made by her childhood friends. The supervising police detective said that originally she accepted the bizarre events described by Diana because they were very believable, complete with specific details. Search warrants were served at her parents' home and those of five families who had been lifelong friends, and police dug up several sites with a backhoe. But in six months of investigation, no supporting evidence was found. The parents were left devastated, unable to comprehend what had happened to them and their daughter. Though Diana had completely cut off any contact with them, she gradually began to question her memories. "I had always called them 'my fantasies' because they felt different, not like the memories I always knew I had. They did feel real, more vivid than my other memories."[6] She came across some articles on False Memory Syndrome and began to wonder if it could have happened to her. A few months later she visited a hypnotherapist. When asked to imagine being downtown on a hot summer day, she was amazed to realize how vivid and real her suggested fantasies could be. The light began to dawn for Diana. If she could create realistic, detailed, and emotionally charged visions with the help of a hypnotherapist, she certainly could do so under the pressure exerted by her therapist and group members. She did the unthinkable—she contacted her parents. She didn't know if it was possible to reconcile, but she wanted to try.

Diana came to me wanting to better understand how she had been pulled into the regression movement and come to believe the things that she had. Step by step, I helped her understand her fantasy-proneness and got her medical help for her recurring depression. With tremendous relief and freedom, Diana came to understand that the images she had fantasized were the product of an active and powerful imagination. Through Project Middle Ground, she was able to reestablish her relationship with her parents, experiencing their forgiveness for the charges she had made. Diana considers it a blessing that her parents were willing to forgive her, but she says, "There will always be scars. It will never be like this never happened."[7]

In the previous two chapters, we examined external influences that can contribute to the development of false memories. But is there something *within* a person that can make her more susceptible to hypnotic fantasies and suggestive therapies? In my work with retractors I've come across a very interesting phenomenon. Like Diana, a number of them describe having strong fantasy abilities throughout their lifetime. It was only when they became involved with regressionism that their fantasy life turned dark and tormented. As an increasing number of retractors confirmed this tendency I began to search for an explanation. My explorations led to two fascinating discoveries: fantasy-prone personalities and Grade five syndrome.

Fantasy-Prone Personalities

In the late 1970s researchers begin to study a segment of the population they described as *fantasy-prone personalities*—people who have a profound ability to fantasize with great detail and emotion, often describing their fantasies as being "as real as real." Importantly, they were *not* mentally disturbed and in fact, appeared to be high-functioning. They had higher education, longstanding marriages, and success in their professions. The researchers estimate that fantasy-prones were possibly 4 percent of the population, predominantly women who fantasized a large portion of the time, even up to 50 percent of their waking day. They could see, hear, smell, touch, and fully experience what they fantasized. In fact, 85 percent of the fantasizers would sometime confuse their memories of fantasies with actual events.[8]

Fantasy-prones demonstrated superb hypnotic performance and could hallucinate voluntarily on request.

The data show hypnotic phenomena are natural for some individuals. Fantasy prone personalities have many experiences throughout their lives that are similar to the classical hypnosis experiences, and they find the suggestions of the hypnotist are very harmonious with their own ongoing experiential life. . . . There are individuals who have a lifetime history of intense fantasy, who have developed hallucinatory abilities, and who—as a result of these talents—are able to quickly, easily, and profoundly experience the classical hypnotic phenomena.[9]

Researchers found a number of interesting details concerning this population:

- They were very secretive about their intense fantasies. Even spouses and best friends had no idea that the fantasy-prone individual had such an intense and expansive fantasy life.
- Fantasies for these individuals often had an involuntary, self-propelling quality. Subjects would notice a person or object around them, which would trigger a long, detailed fantasy.
- They had a tendency toward involvement in psychic experiences, including mystical healings and out-of-body experiences.

Remember that this population is high-functioning and *not* pathological. These people simply represent the far end of the spectrum on the ability to imagine. The researchers note:

A relatively small group of more or less satisfactorily adjusted individuals who live, work, and play like the rest of us, differ from the majority of their fellows, in that, they live much of the time in a world of their own making—in a world of imagery, imagination, and fantasy. They fantasize much of the time when they are not busy; they also fantasize much of the time when they are engaged in relatively non-demanding tasks; and their fantasies tend to become hallucinatory—they are often "as real, as real," and, at times "more real than real."[10]

It was shown that psychologists providing counseling to fantasy-prones had no idea of the special abilities of their clients. In fact, the hypnotic setting provided a situation in which those with a strong, secret fantasy life could publicly demonstrate their special abilities. In hypnosis their ability to fantasize with hallucinatory intensity was not only socially permissible, it was rewarded.

The experiences and behaviors that have been traditionally labeled as hypnotic phenomena are in the repertoire of fantasy prone individuals prior to their having any formal experiences in a hypnosis situation. Hence, when we give them "hypnotic suggestions," such as, suggestions for visual and auditory hallucinations, negative hallucinations, age regression . . . we are asking them to do for us the kind of thing they can do independently of us in their daily lives. However, as we described previously, they have learned to become highly secretive and private about their fantasy life. The hypnosis situation provides them with a social situation which they are encouraged to do, and rewarded for doing, what they usually do only secretly and privately in their fantasy life.[11]

Interestingly, a recent study showed that people who claim to have been space alien abducted are not pathological. But of 152 subjects who claimed space alien abductions and visitations, it was found that 87 percent of them fit the profile for fantasy-prone personality.[12] No study has yet been done on those who claim other forms of recovered memories, but we can assume fantasy-proneness plays an important role in these as well.

Grade Five Syndrome

A closely related concept to fantasy-proneness is the *Grade five syndrome*. Herbert Spiegel, an expert in hypnosis, spent years researching different aspects of hypnotizability. He discovered that 5 to 10 percent of the population was highly hypnotizable: These people he called "Grade five personalities" based on scores on a measure of hypnotizability, called the Hypnotic Induction Profile (HIP).[13] Like the fantasy-prone personalities, the Grade fives are considered "hypnotic virtuosos" who are intellectually and emotionally normal but have an uncanny ability to fantasize. They can spontaneously go into a deep hypnotic trance, even without the aid of a therapist.

Jon Trott, a senior editor at *Cornerstone Magazine*, has written an excellent review of this phenomenon.

Grade fives are particularly vulnerable to something Spiegel calls "the compulsive triad." The first point of the triad, compulsive compliance, is a fancy way of saying that in a trance state fives feel an all-but-overwhelming urge to comply with someone suggesting a new or variant viewpoint. The second leg of the triad, source amnesia, means basically that the five who comes up with certain information is unable to recall where the information actually came from. The third element, rationalization, occurs when the grade five encounters logical opposition to his or her adopted viewpoint.[14]

One can readily see how destructive this process can become when a fantasy-prone personality or a Grade five enters into regression therapy. Trott quotes Sherrill Mulhern, a cult researcher and anthropologist:

Grade fives' highly empathetic abilities make them particularly vulnerable to introspective therapeutic techniques. For example, when they are asked to probe their memories for additional details concerning a particular remembered image or event, Grade fives compulsively respond to their therapists' requests by adding information from various sources into their memories to "fill in the blanks." Researchers found that although these subjects ignore the sources of confabulated details, when questioned about the fallacious information, they make enormous efforts to fit the imagined material logically into the ongoing narrative of their recovered and reexperienced memories.[15]

George Ganaway, director of the Atlanta-based Ridgeview Center for Dissociative Disorders, tested a group of fifty-four patients diagnosed with MPD over a thirty-month period. He reported, "Virtually all of the patients . . . met Spiegel's criteria for the Grade Five Syndrome."[16] Richard Ofshe, an expert on cult dynamics comments on Grade Fives:

Once one misperceives a pseudo-memory as a genuine memory, he now has a basis for believing it has actually happened. And he then becomes a genuine believer in the things that have been "recalled" . . . he's genuinely deceived. Once these themes develop—whatever they are—the consumer of them is really to be pitied. He relies on experts. If those experts pick up on something and start running with it, the receivers have no way of differentiating between truth and falsehood.[17]

Trott warns:

Some therapists use grade fives' testimonies to strengthen their own theories. Others become emotionally involved in grade five stories to the point where objective judgment is lost. Either way, this inappropriate attention motivates the teller to continue to enhance his story. This wide-eyed interest can be enticing for someone who hungers for attention.[18]

Fantasy-prones and Grade fives provide the strongest clues for how healthy people can be pulled into a delusional world of horrific fantasies. Two popular diagnoses that regressionists use with patients are Dissociative Amnesia and Dissociative Identity Disorder (formerly known as Multiple-Personality Disorder, discussed in Chapter 2). The *DSM-IV (Diagnostic and Statistical Manual of Mental Disorders, Fourth Edition)* is the psychological community's official guide for identifying mental disorders. It gives a strong warning about both of these populations.

> Individuals with Dissociative Amnesia often display high hypnotizability as measured by standardized testing. . . . Care must be exercised in evaluating the accuracy of retrieved memories, because the informants are often highly suggestible. There has been considerable controversy concerning amnesia related to reported physical or sexual abuse, particularly when abuse is alleged to have occurred during early childhood. . . . There may be overreporting, particularly given the unreliability of childhood memories. There is currently no method for establishing with certainty the accuracy of such retrieved memories in the absence of corroborative evidence.[19]

The DSM-IV offers a similar caution regarding Dissociative Identity Disorder:

> Controversy surrounds the accuracy of [DID abuse] reports, because childhood memories may be subject to distortion and individuals with this disorder tend to be highly hypnotizable and especially vulnerable to suggestive influences. . . . Individuals with Dissociative Identity Disorder score toward the upper end of the distribution on measures of hypnotizability and dissociative capacity. . . . The syndrome has been overdiagnosed in individuals who are highly suggestible.[20]

There is no evidence that people who undergo real, verified traumas go on to become highly hypnotizable. Real victims of abuse represent the entire spectrum of hypnotizability (all the way from Grade ones to Grade fives). So why is it that people who claim dissociative amnesia and DID highly are hypnotizable? Why are they Grade fives?

As I read the research findings on fantasy-prones and Grade fives, the secrets of the False Memory Crisis were suddenly coming to light. It's not that MPDs and repressed memory victims accidentally happen to be hypnotic virtuosos. It's the other way around—the horse is pulling the cart. Unwitting clients who are highly hypnotizable and suggestible are coming into contact with regressionists and their hypnotic techniques, and, right on cue, are generating the fantasies being suggested to them. In my work with retractors this has certainly proved to be the case. With only the slightest of suggestions, many of the retractors were engaged in creating intensely felt and detailed fantasy traumas. Once their therapists reinforced the hypnotic images as real, the patients were doomed. Trott comments:

> The term "grade five" isn't magic. It isn't some sort of new label to affix on anyone who appears to be gullible. It is an artificial way to describe a real phenomenon. It seems painfully obvious, however, that many of us (including some of evangelism's largest publishers and electronic media outlets) are victimizing highly gullible persons by uncritically repeating sensational testimonial tales.[21]

"I Shall Please"

One of the things I noticed in working with regressed clients was that often there would be an initial improvement in their presenting symptoms after they began experiencing their hypnotic images. They might report a strengthening in their self-esteem, lessening of depression, or relief from chronic pain. These early gains were impressive to me and confirmed that what they were uncovering must be valid. But as therapy continued the "big picture" of their lives deteriorated dramatically until even the initial progress they had made disappeared. I was faced with a dilemma, how could their initial improvements be explained? Why did they eventually disappear?

Science has discovered a fascinating principle called the *placebo effect*, which is Latin for "I shall please." A large portion of people can experience physical and psychological relief from painful symptoms simply by taking an innocuous sugar pill or engaging in a non-sensical procedure. The key is that the person believes that the pill or procedure has a healing effect, a process that is referred to as the "power of suggestion." With sincere belief the mind takes over and natural healing processes are engaged. In his book *Pain The Gift Nobody Wants*,[22] Paul Brand, a physician, notes the powerful effects of placebos and suggestion. In one study cancer patients reported substantial relief from pain after placebo treatments. Some were given placebo pills, others had placebo shots, and a third group had intravenous placebo drips. In each case the patients reported improvements, with the intravenous drip showing the strongest improvement (50 percent). Some of the patients even had withdrawal symptoms after the treatment was halted. But the pills, shots and drips were fakes, they had no scientific properties that would produce therapeutic benefit. In another experiment, done in 1939, doctors conducted heart surgeries on a group of patients. Half of them had an actual medical procedure done but the other half were simply put under general anesthesia, had their chests cut open and then promptly sewn up. Post-surgery both groups of patients showed comparable improvements—their pain diminished, they took less medication, and could exercise more.

There are volumes of studies which demonstrate the placebo effect and help explain why it is that people can experience healing when given non-scientific procedures or believe in superstitious practices. The initial relief I was seeing in my own clients was simply an example of the placebo effect in action. The official-sounding pronouncements, the money, time, sincere beliefs, and effort to find meaning to their problems provided the motivation for clients to believe in the healing powers of regressionism. But the initial benefits they were experiencing were only temporary. Clients were actually given a false hope at the start, which led them even deeper into a regression belief system. As they slipped further in, the placebos' effects wore off and were gradually replaced by psychotic decompensation as they moved further away from reality.

Personality Types

How sickness enlarges the dimensions of a man's self to himself! He is his own exclusive object. Supreme selfishness is inculcated upon him as his only duty.
CHARLES LAMB, *THE CONVALESCENT*, 1833

The good news is that regression clients are increasingly finding their way back to reality. These retractors are coming out after years of regression involvement with astounding loss: destroyed families, divorces, lost careers, multiple suicide attempts, massive debt, and the aftereffects of toxic group involvement. When I asked them how they got out, they often point to different things that disrupted the "closed system" of their regression mindset, i.e., running out of insurance, moving to a different city, or a family crisis. Many just got tired. The regression promises turned into years of disappointment and increasing self-deterioration. Whether through disruption or fatigue, these clients were finally able to begin asking forbidden questions about their therapies. The answers they discovered led them back to truth and away from the deception they had been inducted into. Once out, the retractors typically were furious about their therapeutic torture and seeking justice. Our study in 1993 showed that 63 percent of retractors were litigating against their regressionists for different aspects of malpractice.[23]

But if it's simply a matter of someone understanding that she's been tricked into believing hypnotic fantasies, how is it that some people are coming out while others choose to stay in their delusions? With such painful, devastating results in their lives, why don't all of them become retractors? The answer lies in some of the dynamics we've already explored: a victim's paradigm, toxic-group coercion, double-binding, threats, emotional investment, brief reactive psychosis, and resulting paranoid delusional disorders. But my work with regression believers has also revealed a core drive within some to stay in the victim's role. Unlike retractors who found their way back out, I found that many clients who remained in regressionism were actually excited to uncover their hidden traumas and delighted in going into great detail about their victimization. They basked in the attention and pity that they received from myself, other therapists, and group members. Astonishingly, they found a great deal of pleasure and benefit in their role as victims, in sharp contrast to my work with victims of actual abuse who had always remembered their trauma. Is it possible that someone can actually want to play out the victim's role? The answer lies in understanding personality disorders.

Each of us has certain tendencies in our thinking and behavior that are characteristic of who we are. "He's a studious and serious person." "She's easygoing and fun to be with." Psychologists refer to strong characteristics as *personality types* which reflect enduring patterns of how a person perceives and relates to others, his environment, and self. These personality types are exhibited in a wide range of social situations and cross the span of a person's life. Sometimes a personality type becomes inflexible and maladaptive and can cause significant personal and relational problems. When this happens, psychologists refer to these rigid types as *personality disorders.*

Personality Disorders

"Andrea" has been in regression therapy for four and a half years and has been diagnosed with multiple personalities. Her hypnotic fantasies include being raised in a multigenerational satanic cult, having borne three babies that were sacrificed by the cult, and having survived numerous cult rituals involving drinking blood and urine, multiple rapes, and killings. On one occasion she even recalls being encased in the empty carcass of a dead wolf and being "reborn" as a bride of Satan who had been chosen to be the next high priestess. Currently she has a colorful menagerie of different alters, including a giggling little girl, an erotic lesbian, three demons, four men of varying temperaments, a dog, a destructive persona named Dark Man, and twelve other personalities. She is convinced that cult members still follow her around day and night, listen in on all her phone conversations, and secretly enter into her home and office when she is away. This is because they want her to come back to the cult as their chosen leader. Meanwhile, she occasionally cuts herself with razors and burns herself with matches or cigarettes and has been in psychiatric hospitals for four extended stays. Each time she stabilizes and comes back into the caring arms of her therapist and recovery group. She sees her therapist, Larry, twice a week and attends three different support groups weekly. She credits each of them with having saved her life on many occasions, unlike her ex-husband who just didn't seem to understand her needs.

She is attending her third church in as many years. Caring Christians have her hidden in a "safe house" in the hopes that the satanists won't find her. She has created quite a commotion at the church, with constant accusations that different Christian leaders and local church members are members of the cult. She is often at odds with different people because they fail to appreciate the immense danger and pain that she is in. "So many people can't even comprehend how difficult life is for me. To have the terrifying memories, to be followed by evil forces constantly. They just don't understand. They're just not safe for me. That's why I have to establish a boundary to keep them at a safe distance until they accept my reality without questioning it."[24]

There's a bit of a problem in all this. Her fantasies aren't true. Extensive police investigations and evidence produced by family and friends conclusively prove her stories are fraudulent. But in today's victim-affirming, witch-hunt atmosphere, Andrea is able to find a large audience that will attend to her every claim without question. Her real issues are actually much less exotic. Andrea's story, repeated in thousands of other regression clients, captures the essence of borderline, paranoid, and narcissistic personality disorders.

Borderline Personality

"Andrea's" violent temper, relational extremes, constant fear of abandonment, and self-destructive behaviors are mislabeled as symptoms of MPD, but in reality they're simply the product of a common disorder, borderline personality. The symptoms include instability in relationships, uncertain self-image, efforts to avoid real or imagined abandonment, alternating between idealizing and then devaluating others, destructive impulses, recurrent suicidal behaviors, inappropriate anger, and stress-related paranoid beliefs.

For a borderline personality like Andrea, repressed traumas are a perfect explanation for why she has these problems. This explanation casts the blame for Andrea's behavior on someone else— there is nothing she has to be responsible for. Every lost relationship, every time she cuts herself, every church she leaves in complete chaos is not her fault: It's her murderous, multigenerational satanist daddy's fault. In fact, she is given cart blanche to act out in any way she feels like, because she is a "heroic survivor" and now is her chance to live out the childhood she was denied.

Paranoid Personality

With the aid of hypnosis and the encouragement of her therapist, Andrea was able to create vivid fantasies of murderous satanists who were everywhere and manipulating day-to-day events in an effort to harm her. Her descent into regressionism is in harmony with her preexisting paranoid personality. Paranoid personalities are generally functional and selectively reality-based in their perceptions, but as is the case with Andrea, if their paranoia is fed it expands to increasingly grotesque proportions. Symptoms include distrusting others, interpreting other's motives as being malevolent, preoccupation with doubts about friends' loyalty, reluctance to confide in others, reading hidden meanings in benign remarks, and being unforgiving.

Narcissistic Personality

This personality type demonstrates a triad of vanity, exhibitionism, and arrogant ingratitude that involves an overall preoccupation with one's self. The narcissist often has delusions of grandeur in which he or she holds a very special role. Interestingly, when I'm talking with SRA "survivors" they typically declare that they are the next "high priestess" of their satanic cult. By imagining she is a high priestess who is desperately struggling to free herself from the clutches of powerful cult members who want to worship her, Andrea and other narcissists are able to turn a mundane, ordinary world into one of excitement, where they play center stage in a cosmic battle. The voracious appetite of the narcissist is able to find daily sustenance from the therapeutic community that promotes "self" as the ultimate goal. Anyone who fails to attend to the narcissist's endless needs is deemed a threat and leads to an emotional explosion on the narcissist's part. On the other hand, anyone who provides constant positive acceptance and encouragement, even in the face of non-reality, is seen as "good."

Histrionic Personality Disorder

When "Alice" walks into a room, everyone notices. She always dresses in a colorful, bright fashion, tends to gush all sorts of emotions, and talks as if people are a bit deaf. It seems like her life is one long series of disappointments and tragedies. Six months ago she started regression therapy and the drama has exploded hundredfold. Now every Thursday night at her church community group she tearfully describes how she is discovering an ever-expanding litany of horrible abuses. "Please pray for me. The truths I'm rediscovering are devastating."[25] Alice demonstrates the common traits of the histrionic, which includes excessive emotionalism, attention-seeking, a desire to be the center of attention, shallow expression of feelings, a physical appearance that draws attention, over-dramatic speech and conduct, and being very suggestible.

Notice that this personality trait is closely related to borderline personality, but is not as debilitating. Regression therapy provides the perfect theatrical stage for the histrionic. Egged on by the regressionist and group members, she is able to be the constant center of attention, be sexually explicit with others under the guise of "being honest in therapy," and wildly dramatic—crying, screaming, acting like a little child. Twenty years ago, a therapist would have told her grow up and take responsibility for herself, but today's regressionist will tell her to "get into your inner child and allow complete freedom of expression"—an absolute disaster.

Obsessive-Compulsive Personality

This is a workaholic type who is perfectionistic and driven. He tends to be overconscientious, self-sacrificing, and hardworking. In healthy balance, the obsessive-compulsive is a productive and conscientious worker. But in extreme this person becomes incapable of relaxing and is focused on pleasing others and working too much, and he or she has trouble handling emotions. When I'm doing a seminar with accused families I'll often ask, "How many here consider your accusing daughter or son to be a high achiever—she or he had straight As in school, completed college and graduate studies, were perfectionistic?" Consistently, 60 to 70 percent of the families raise their hands and they experience a moment of discovery.

Think about this for a moment. As we've already discussed, sexual abuse and tortures do not enhance a child's academic performance. It actually affects it in a seriously adverse manner. Yet many of the regression believers that I've talked to can point to stellar academic and professional achievements—the exact opposite of what we would expect to find.

The obsessive-compulsive personality type gives us some clues. Common sense tells us that people who are tuned to what those in authority expect are the ones that maintain straight As in school and jump all the hurdles just right. It's a matter of correctly reading expectations and working hard at meeting and pleasing. An obsessive-compulsive does this for years. She gets all the right degrees and promotions—the perfect student and employee. These are the same personality characteristics she carries into therapy, where a person in authority reveals to her the "real" nature of her problems. She is told that if she applies herself diligently and does not resist the therapeutic process, she will come into greater wholeness than she has ever known. As the hypnotic images begin to come, she is praised and encouraged by her therapist, the very pattern that the client has followed throughout her life.

Dependent Personality

"Sally" has always had a poor self-image. She lacks confidence, is soft-spoken, and never likes making her own decisions. She got into a marriage in which her husband had become increasingly controlling and abusive, but she simply didn't have the strength to take a stand against his cruel treatment. In desperation she turned to therapy. The relief she found was tremendous. Her regressionist helped her understand why she had always been this way, that she's acting out secret abuses she had repressed. Sally learned to trust her regressionist completely, following his every directive. As the weeks turned into months, she became increasingly dependent and devoted, little by little giving all control over to him.

Dependent personalities are one of the most frequently reported disorders in counseling centers. Their symptoms include a constant need to be taken care of, submissive and clinging behaviors, fear of separation, difficulty making everyday decisions without excessive advice, fear of disagreeing with others, lacking independent initiative, going to great lengths to get support from others, and fear of being left alone. In the context of regressionism, this personality type is quickly pulled into a destructive dependency on her therapist.

Borderline, narcissistic, histrionic, and so on—psychologists have discovered personality disorders are tenacious and resistant to change. They are common, time-consuming, and difficult to treat. The therapist who simply sits down and listens, hypnotizes, and encourages the narcissist, borderline, or histrionic to go with her thoughts and feelings is throwing fuel on the fire of the disorder. By misdiagnosing, the therapists are exacerbating the personality disorder rather than providing the proper treatment: a structured and accountable intervention, with a "here and now" focus. Diagnosis is everything. Before we can ever begin treatment, we must first know what we're treating. Imagine if a person went into a physician's office with a broken toe and his presenting aliment was misdiagnosed as stemming from a brain tumor. The physician happened to be a brain tumor specialist and the subsequent operation was performed flawlessly. He earned $48,000 for doing the brain operation, compared to the seventy dollars he would have earned to fix a broken toe. But in the end, the toe still isn't fixed and the patient has lost half of his cerebral cortex in the process. Truth matters. Getting the right diagnosis—before treatment—matters.

For some of the regression believers I spoke with I could tell their personality disorders had been in place long before their journey into regressionism. But for others, including most of the retractors, I discovered they only developed severe personality changes once they had entered regressionism, like the radical personality shifts researchers see in new cult members. The good news is that personality disorders that are a by-product of regression therapy are quickly relieved once the client is able to escape her therapist. Pamela Freyd, of the FMS Foundation, notes:

A legal suit brought by a retractor against her therapist . . . was settled in spring of 1995 in favor of the retractor. The suit was brought in King County Superior Court of Washington and evidence was introduced that noted that the patient had tested in the normal range on a standard personality test at the beginning of therapy. Her test results were elevated well beyond normal limits after therapy began and hypnosis was used. The patient did appear to have suffered severe trauma, but the trauma seems to have taken place in the therapy.[26]

Effort After Meaning

On a number of occasions I've encountered regression believers who had serious psychological disorders—schizophrenia, clinical depression, anxiety disorders or panic attacks, which were clearly evident before they began their regression therapy. They came to regressionism desperate for answers to their pain, hoping for some cure, and the sure-sounding theories of the regressionist promised relief. But rather than getting better, clients' disorders grew worse. All the while convinced that their healing was just around the corner—a few recovered memories away. But the promised healing simply was not forthcoming.

During my early years of training as a psychologist I was taught an interesting and popular theory. Experts believed that schizophrenia was the result of a person growing up in a dysfunctional home. It was theorized that the parents engaged in a process called *double binding*, in which two conflicting messages were being given to a child ("I'm torturing you because I love you."). The resulting schizophrenia was due to the child's splitting in order to be able to accept both contradictory messages. Tragically, for several decades double binding was a popular belief in the psychological community. Fortunately, with the progression of time and science, we've since been able to understand this is not the case. Schizophrenia is a physical disorder—there are no parents to blame. But can you imagine the indescribable pain of thousands of parents over those decades? Not only did they have a child who was acting in bizarre, self-destructive ways, to further complicate things the parents were told that they were to blame for their child's illness.

Notions such as "double binding" reflect an ongoing problem in psychology. "Witch-hunting," back then and in the present, holds to a common and primitive thinking—if something is wrong with a person then there must be someone else to blame. As with the myth of double binding, therapists continue to blame parents for a wide variety of mental disorders. Please don't misunderstand, in some instances parents can play a direct role in difficulties a child experiences. But clearly many therapists have gone overboard in their blaming. The question is, "Why does witch-hunting continue to have such appeal in our culture?"

In science we talk about a process called *effort after meaning*. All of us are prone to make sense out of tragic events that befall others or ourselves. If someone we love dies or if we discover that we have a serious physical disorder, we make a strong *effort* to find *meaning* in the situation. Those with mental and emotional pain are no different—"If I can discover who caused this depression, then I'll be cured." "Tell me someone else is to blame, that it's not me that is defective." Think about this for a moment. If you were a schizophrenic, would you rather live with the reality of the diagnosis or would you prefer to be told you were a bold survivor of horrific abuses? That your mental disorder was actually a coping mechanism which had allowed you to survive your abusers' assaults? Promised that if you could unlock the deadly secrets inside of you, then and only then could you come to know true relief from your agony. Tell me, which diagnosis would you choose?

"Effort after meaning" helps explain the earlier witch-hunts in which a tragedy was thought to be somebody's evil doing. These same primitive superstitions are embodied at the heart of regressionism. If you're depressed, have anxiety, any disorder under the sun—some evil person is the cause of it. The truth is that physical and mental illness happens for lots of people. It's a reality that is part of a fallen creation.

Meanwhile, the implications are overwhelming. Not only have reasonably healthy people been taken in by regressionism, but the mentally and emotionally ill, who are most vulnerable to fraud and manipulation, have been duped into believing regression's claims. Who stands in the gap to protect them from these abuses? At the moment, no one.

The Blame Game

There's a common variation of "effort after meaning" that we all contend with. And you don't need a mental disorder in order to play it. From the first chapters of our creation we have a demonstrated tendency to "pass the buck" when it comes to taking responsibility for our own bad choices. In Genesis, Adam and Eve were given complete freedom to eat from any tree in the garden. There was only one restriction—they were not to eat of the tree of the knowledge of good and evil. Which is, of course, what they proceeded to do. When confronted, Adam's response is to blame God and Eve—*"The woman you put here with me—she gave me some fruit from the tree, and I ate it."* In turn, Eve blames the serpent— *"The serpent deceived me, and I ate."* One gets the idea that the fruit got down off the tree all by itself, walked over to Adam and Eve and leapt into their unwilling mouths.

We've been remarkably good students in learning from their example and have excelled in the "blame game." The recovered memory movement in modern America is a sterling example of victim culture at its very worst. The pain of being overweight, in a bad marriage, addicted to alcohol, lazy, and a legion of other consequences from wrong choices are conveniently blamed on fantasies of abusing satanists, space aliens, or parents, rather then the logical result of inappropriate decisions a person has made. If Adam and Eve had parents, you can bet that a regression therapist would have uncovered the true reason for their poor choices.

The point is this—each of us possess within us the free will to choose life or death. Every single day you and I make choices. Some good, some bad. They're our choices and we're responsible for the consequences. But the recovered memory movement offers a tempting fruit that calls to one of our deepest vices— blame. It's "effort after meaning" with a twist. The recovered "meaning" absolves us of taking responsibility for our own poor choices.

Points to Remember

Internal generation of false memories can be influenced by a variety of factors. These include:

✓ *Fantasy Prone Personalities* are high-functioning people and estimated to be 4 percent of the population. These individuals fantasize a large part of the time, can "see, hear, smell, touch, and fully experience what they fantasize," and provide superb hypnotic performances. The danger is that these healthy individuals are highly suggestible and can experience traumatic fantasies that feel real.

✓ Those with *Grade Five Syndrome* are very similar to Fantasy Prone Personalities and are considered to be "hypnotic virtuosos," intellectually and emotionally normal but have an uncanny ability to fantasize. They can spontaneously go into a deep hypnotic trance, even without the aid of a therapist. They are noted for their compulsive compliance, source amnesia, and rationalizations.

✓ The *Placebo Effect* helps to explain how some people can experience initial improvement in regression therapy. But these early gains are short-lived as the destructive processes of regressionism continue.

✓ There are unhealthy internal states which can also contribute to the generation of false memories. These include *Borderline, Paranoid, Narcissistic, Histrionic, Obsessive-Compulsive,* and *Dependent* personality disorders which find tremendous secondary gain in the role of "victim."

✓ Those with clinical disorders like *depression, schizophrenia,* or *anxiety* are particularly susceptible to the influences of regression doctrine because it provides hope, *"effort after meaning"* and they are most vulnerable to manipulation and false information.

✓ The *"blame game"* appeals to a natural desire to avoid taking responsibility for our own poor choices.

11

Angels of Light? The Spiritual Question

For our struggle is not against flesh and blood, but against the rulers, against the authorities, against the powers of this dark world and against the spiritual forces of evil in the heavenly realms.

EPHESIANS 6:12

"Joe" and "Alice" are parents of three children and grandparents to seven grandchildren. Devoted Christians throughout their lives, they had raised their children with a respect and knowledge of God. With a look of embarrassment, Joe hands me a letter they received from their youngest daughter. Like thousands of other families, their daughter sent them a "confrontation letter" that reveals the content of the hypnotic images the daughter has experienced. The letter bears the classic hallmarks of someone caught up in regressionism. Notice the use of a little girl's wording and voice, and her use of "we" in describing herself and her many "alter personalities" she discovered in therapy. (Explicit language has been deleted.)

Dear Mother and Father,

I know you have been wondering why I've broken contact with you. This letter will explain everything. The rest of the family will also know because I am sending copies to them. I've often wondered why I act like an adult one minute and a child the next. Well, the answer is I've been diagnosed as having Multiple Personality Disorder (MPD). I have MPD because of what you both did to me as a child. We needed to create others so we could grow up.

We're not crazy. You see we've begun to remember. You had no right to do what you did. There were times we wanted to kill both of you. You will never convince us that we are wrong. You see, we know the truth. The fantasy is over and we live in reality now. We realize we never had a mom and dad and never will. We're not sure about putting some of the details in but we've decided to do it. This is probably going to gross you out. I know it did me when my alters gave me the information.

179

Mother, when we were three years old you taped our ankles and hung us upside down. You did it again and again for many years. You also pour[ed] bugs on us. We were naked. You didn't believe us when we [were] real little and tried to tell you what father was making us do. You let the head of the cult do bad things to us. You touched us and let others touch us. . . .

Father, you never did stop sexually abusing us until the day we moved out. It started in the crib. . . . You kept raping us until we were an adult, even up to two and a half years ago. I never knew that until the alters let me know. You were always walking into our room and bathroom while we showered. We couldn't sleep naked for fear of you walking in the next morning. You made sexual comments to us or even women in general.

Both of you involved us in the cult when we were four. We sure . . . didn't want to believe it. Especially, with the things they made us do. You held our hands over a knife and killed some cats while other man caught the blood in some type of white bowls. You see we were too little to hold the knife by ourselves. You convinced us that we were doing the killing. You painted us with some of the blood. And made us drink it too. When we were older you told us "Kill or be killed." So we killed the baby. Again someone caught all the blood then the man in charge cut out the heart. He put it in the bowl of blood. Then he held it up and blessed it. He chanted something while he painted me with some of the blood. He made me eat some of the heart and drink some of the blood. He also cut off its head. When we were littler he [was] the one to kill the baby. He does the same stuff to it and to us. You and mother . . . should never been allowed to have kids.

We're taking control back. From this day forward I stop acknowledging you as mom and dad. I will accept no gifts from either of you. I will not be bought. None of us will. Also to make it complete I will legally be changing my name. For your information we broke up with Michael because we are lesbian. There, we're glad that secret's out too. Also, we know we have more to remember but we are on that road to recovery. This has been a big step for us.

Hate You Always,
Susan

Did "Susan" really forget all these horrible events? Were these true memories that her different "personalities" revealed to her? Are the various lesbians, men, animals, and children that she has discovered inside of her authentic and a part of her "road to recovery"? Could they be the creation of her own twisted mind? Or, is it possible that her destructive, raging personalities serve a greater purpose and point us to another influence?

In the last three chapters we've discussed possible external and internal contributors to false memories. As a psychologist, I realize the importance of examining the False Memory Crisis in the light of science and reason, and I believe that much of what we've discussed can be understood through natural processes. However, I also recognize that science has limits regarding how far it can go in identifying and explaining reality, that there are important theological and philosophical spheres science simply cannot examine. You see, psychology is something I do as a profession, something that I enjoy a great deal. But Christian is what I am, who I belong to, the paradigm that most accurately defines my worldview. My faith as a Christian calls me to take one step further in my quest to understand, to see the "big picture," one which encompasses physical and spiritual reality. In this chapter I want to address the False Memory Crisis from the Christian perspective.

A Christian since 1972, I've always been active in my faith. I became involved in the charismatic movement in the mid-seventies and eventually graduated from Bethany College, an Assemblies of God school in California, with majors in biblical studies and psychology. Through the years I've worked with various Christian organizations, including Teen Challenge, Campus Crusade for Christ, and Rapha (a Christian inpatient treatment program). In those years and experiences I have discovered many good things about the Christian community. But I have also been a part of incredible excesses, a process that I call "ignorance on fire." At various times I've watched myself and other believers zealously convinced that we were engaged in a mighty work of God, when in fact we were simply in a flat-out silly pursuit (see Prov. 19:2).

In C. S. Lewis's book, *The Screwtape Letters*, the Senior devil (Screwtape) advises his junior devil:

> What we want, if men become Christians at all, is to keep them in the state of mind I call "Christianity And." You know—Christianity and the Crisis, Christianity and the New Psychology, Christianity and the New Order, Christianity and Faith Healing, Christianity and Psychical Research, Christianity and Vegetarianism, Christianity and Spelling Reform. If they must be Christians, let them at least be Christians with a differ-

ence. Substitute for the faith itself some Fashion with a Christian colouring. Work on their horror of the Same Old Thing.[1]

True to form, many of us have come to embrace the deception of "Christianity And"—Christianity and the fight against multigenerational satanists, Christianity and self-actualization, Christianity and recovered memories. In this chapter I pursue the most difficult questions I've yet asked in my quest to understand the False Memory Crisis. A few years ago I would have been very offended if someone suggested that my clients' recovered memories were a product of misdirected therapy. But I would have been outraged if they said my work was deceptive and in opposition to God's purposes. I truly believed that God was active in the work that I was doing. Through His leading and sincerity on my part, I believed I was unlocking hidden secrets in clients' lives. But truth matters, regardless of how sincere an advocate is or politically expedient his conclusion. In the final analysis we must ask, "Is it true?"

The Christian Faith Confronts the Recovered Memory Movement

"A religion that is jealous of the variety of learning, discourse, opinions, and sects, as misdoubting it may shake the foundations, or that cherisheth devotion upon simplicity and ignorance, as ascribing ordinary effects to the immediate working of God, is adverse to knowledge."
SIR FRANCIS BACON, OF THE INTERPRETATION OF NATURE

Steve, a Christian therapist, practices regressionism in a large, conservative church in the Southwest. In his brand of regression, clients are told they have symptoms that indicate repressed memories of sexual and ritual abuse and to ask God what happened to them. "We tell a person to get a private place, and prior to sitting down, ask God to reveal anything about her relationship with her father that she may have repressed or forgotten about. We have the belief that God does, in fact, answer prayers.... If I ask God to guide my thoughts, I believe that what comes into my mind should be taken on faith."[2]

In this self-induced hypnotic state, the client inevitably generates the traumatic images that have been suggested to her. When she returns and says "God told me I was sexually abused by my parents," that's enough evidence for Steve. As far as he's concerned, no further investigation is needed. He concedes clients may, in fact, simply imagine that God is answering their prayers. But unless they have a history of exaggeration or report being told something "that God wouldn't say," the content of their conversations is taken on faith.

> It comes down to whether you're going to trust your patients. Is there anything to do but trust them? Not really. If you come across as disbelieving, what you've done psychologically is to revictimize them. . . . The point is that they sincerely believe these things happened to them, and they are traumatized by that belief. Our job is to help that person, not to play detective. . . . It's not our job to try to find out the truth.[3]

I met with Steve and his counseling staff one afternoon, hoping I could persuade them to become more aware of the dangers of their rationalizations and practices. We had a polite and informative conversation, and I found them to be very sincere in their convictions about regressionism, just as I was at one time. They truly believed that there is no need to verify the accusations against other people, as long as the victim sincerely believes her hypnotic fantasies to be true. They were appreciative that I took the time to meet with them, but they explained that these were spiritually discerned matters. All the research findings I had discussed with them didn't apply because this was a "work of the Holy Spirit." Unfortunately, their response echoes a common zeal that I encounter with Christian regressionists.

When I set out to discover the truth about regressionism, I sought to apply two different tests for its validity. The first test was scientific, called *general revelation*, and the second was biblical, called *special revelation*. General revelation is the idea that there are truths revealed to us through God's created order that aren't necessarily talked about in Scripture (see Rom. 1:20). Meanwhile, special revelation (sometimes called higher revelation) relates to those truths that come to us through the Scriptures. Truth found in general revelation is complementary to special revelation and vice versa. There is a harmony found between the two, and each elaborates on the other.

Early in my search to better understand my regression beliefs and practices, I knew there wasn't any biblical support (special revelation) for my position. But I figured that it could still be true because it was scientific (general revelation). "Repressed memo-

ries and regression techniques are scientific realities! Even though
the Bible doesn't mention them, it doesn't mean they aren't real!
Lots of scientific discoveries aren't noted in the Bible, but they're
part of God's created order nonetheless. Just because the atomic
bomb and the polio vaccine aren't named in Scripture doesn't
mean they don't exist."

But there's a problem with this line of thinking. Atomic bombs
and polio vaccines are scientific fact, open to verification by anyone. But in sharp contrast, my search revealed that regressionism
was anything but scientific. This is what we discussed in the first
half of this book. Regression theory is not scientifically valid and
regression techniques constitute mental-health fraud. On the first
test, regressionism fails God's general revelation.

But what about the other test, special revelation? For Christian
regressionists an important underlying assumption is that regression theory and practice are biblical truths that we have uncovered
in these latter times (special revelation). Maybe I was too quick in
discounting this as a work of the Holy Spirit. Perhaps regressionism is a spiritually discerned matter, a biblical truth that I've over-
looked? And how about this new gifting of the Holy Spirit, in
which He suddenly starts taking believers back in time to unlock
forgotten memories of ritual abuse, incest, and former lives? The
Bible describes so many marvelous gifts of the Spirit. Surely God's
Word would have something to say about this new, powerful gifting! Somewhere it must say that in the end times the Holy Spirit
will come upon believers and reveal to them hidden abuses. So I
turn to the Bible and find. . . silence.

Is it possible that God forgot to tell us that in the latter days the
Holy Spirit would have this special gift for us, fail to even mention
how to access this powerful, revelational work? Historically the
Christian community has always pressed forward to a higher standard in our search for truth. For us the bottom line for any belief
or practice is, "Is this in harmony with the Word of God [special
revelation]?" Amazingly, we have abandoned this standard when
it comes to the subject of regression theories. This much we know
for sure, regressionism is not a doctrine taught anywhere in the
Bible. Nowhere are we instructed to pursue forgotten memories.
Nowhere is the Holy Spirit described as a memory aid for forgotten abuses, mythical satanists, or prior lives. There is no evidence
in Church history that the Holy Spirit has ever unlocked hidden
traumatic memories in a believer.

In justifying their practices, Christian regression believers inevitably quote to me John 8:32, "Then you will know the truth, and the truth will set you free." But they always fail to mention the first half of this Scripture. Christ said, "If you hold to my teaching, you are really my disciples. Then you will know the truth, and the truth will set you free" (John 8:31–32 NIV). Nowhere in any of Christ's teaching is recovery of forgotten memories implied or taught. It is only as we come to embrace Christ and His teachings, His truth, that we come to know true freedom. So whose "truth" are regressionists referring to? Regressionism, a Freudian belief system, emphasizes that its disciples must live with a backward focus, spending years and vast amounts of time and money in search of hidden incest, prior lives, or space alien memories that are suspected to have occurred decades or centuries ago. Once these hypnotic images are experienced the client gives them center stage in her life, is never allowed to question their reality, and descends into an ever darker stairway of rage, bitterness, selfishness, hate, and isolation.

In sharp contrast, Scripture teaches a forward-looking focus: "But one thing I do: Forgetting what is behind and straining toward what is ahead, I press on toward the goal to win the prize for which God has called me heavenward in Christ Jesus" (Phil. 3:13–14). As we live out Christ's truth, we naturally bear fruit of "love, joy, peace, longsuffering, kindness, goodness, faithfulness, gentleness, self-control" (Gal. 5:22–23). Believers learn to value others as greater than themselves and their lives reflect service and sacrifice. Paul challenges us, "Do not conform any longer to the pattern of this world, but be transformed by the renewing of your mind. Then you will be able to test and approve what God's will is—his good, pleasing and perfect will" (Rom. 12:2 NIV). Regression disciples allow themselves to become enslaved to their own horrific thoughts, engrossed in each sordid detail. But Christ's teachings and truth are diametrically opposed to these beliefs and practices. Philippians 4:7–8 offer a marvelous promise:

> And the peace of God, which transcends all understanding, will guard your hearts and minds in Christ Jesus. Finally, brothers, whatever is true, whatever is noble, whatever is right, whatever is pure, whatever is lovely, whatever is admirable—if anything is excellent or praiseworthy—think about such things. (NIV)

In 2 Corinthians 10:5 we are told to "take captive every thought to make it obedient to Christ." A retractor I worked with summed it up beautifully: "For me, the lesson I would offer my therapist and everyone else who believes in regression therapy is this: God didn't say 'Renew your feelings,' He said 'Renew your mind.' He didn't say 'Take every feeling captive,' He said 'Take every thought captive.'"[4]

How is it that the Holy Spirit had to wait two thousand years, until the advent of Sigmund Freud, before this particular gift could be introduced to the Christian community? Is it possible that the Holy Spirit has not blessed the beliefs and practices of the Christian regressionists? Could it be that all we've done within Christian therapy is mimic the world's latest craze? Did we sprinkle "Jesus pixie dust" on dangerous practices and believe that it somehow sanctified and authenticated this pursuit?

In the final analysis, my search for truth revealed that regression doctrine and practice fail on both tests of validity. They are not shown to be scientific (God's general revelation) and they are not shown to be biblical (God's special revelation).

"Is the regressionists' use of 'Holy Spirit guides' really different from hypnosis?"

"There is a sort of transcendental ventriloquy through which men can be made to believe that something which was said on earth came from heaven."
GEORG CHRISTOPH LICHTENBERG, *APHORISMS*, 1764–99

In my conversations with Steve and his regression team, they assured me that they didn't use hypnosis. Regardless of Scripture's silence, they believed what they were doing was a work of the Holy Spirit. Christian regressionists always confidently inform me that they don't use hypnosis to unlock repressed memories in their clients. They're very aware that hypnosis has a bad reputation within the Christian community. But when I ask them how they unlock memories in their clients, they invariably describe the following scenario. First they have the client close her eyes, and then empty herself of any distracting thoughts or images. The regressionist then prays that the "Holy Spirit" will come upon the person and take her back in time to unlock forgotten traumas. Remember Steve's version, "We tell a person to get to a private place, and prior to sitting down, ask God to reveal anything about her relationship with her father that she may have repressed or forgotten about." With the "Holy Spirit's" help, the client is able to see the horrific truths she has repressed for so long, and everyone can be assured that the images are true because the "Holy Spirit" has blessed the entire proceedings.

Time for a reality check. This is a description of hypnosis, plain and simple. It involves the same standard induction steps that allow a person to move into a relaxed state of trance. In this highly suggestible, fantasizing state, the client is then able to produce the fantasies that have been suggested to her by her therapist, group members, and readings. It is, of course, a far cry from any kind of biblical understanding of the Holy Spirit's role in our life. As we discussed, nowhere in God's Word is it even remotely implied that the Holy Spirit can be used as a spirit guide to bring us to repressed memories. But by relabeling hypnotic trance techniques "Holy Spirit guidance," Christian regressionists have misled clients to believe that they were not engaging in hypnosis when in fact they were.

Let's be clear: You can call hypnotic trance "age regression," "Holy Spirit guidance," "New Age Spirit guides," "a plate of spaghetti," whatever you want. But calling this rose by another name does not remove its thorns. The reality is that the Christian regressionist and client are not engaging in an act of faith, what they're doing is classic hypnotic trance. All the dangers and limitations of hypnosis that we've discussed in previous chapters still apply.

"Does the Bible teach that prayer will automatically protect us from any harm or deception?"

Steve explained, "We have the belief that God does, in fact, answer prayers. . . . If I ask God to guide my thoughts, I believe that what comes into my mind should be taken on faith." A number of Christian regressionists I have talked with agree with this view. They sincerely believe that God answers prayer and that whatever comes into a person's mind after such a prayer should be taken on faith as being real. This is something that I was in complete agreement with a few years ago. But think for a moment. This is a very important assumption. Does prayer automatically protect us from harm, regardless of what we're engaging in?

First of all, we need to recognize the difference between magical thinking and Christian faith. Unfortunately, some Christians view God as a great big "rabbit's foot" in the sky: If you hold Him real, real tight, and believe with all your heart and remove any doubts, then you'll be safe from any harm, regardless of what you're doing. Remember Gale in Chapter 4? She assured me that she knew that her prior life was real because the "Holy Spirit" had revealed it to her after a great deal of prayer. Superstitions, even with Christian trappings, are still superstitions.

Time for another reality check. Prayer doesn't bless or promise safe passage for an immoral pursuit. Scripture warns us about those who have turned their hearts away from God and have followed other gods, "He blesses himself in his heart, saying, 'I shall have peace, even though I walk in the imagination of my heart'" (Deut. 29:19 KJV). Simply put, the prayer the regressionist refers to is not prayer directed in God's Word, but rather something he uses as a "lucky charm" for engaging in dangerous practices. This much we know for sure, God is not a puppet on a string, blindly granting us our every wish. Prayer isn't a magical incantation that automatically protects a person from foolish choices.

When Satan was tempting Jesus at the top the temple and he encouraged Him to throw Himself down so that angels would save Him, Jesus responded, "Do not put the Lord your God to the test" (Matt. 4:7 NIV). Paul warns us, "See to it that no one takes you captive through hollow and deceptive philosophy, which depends on human tradition and the basic principles of this world rather than on Christ" (Col. 2:8 NIV). As we discussed in Chapter 8, hypnosis involves giving up one's ability for critical discernment and opening up to vivid fantasies and suggestions. In contrast, God's Word warns us to "...take captive every thought to make it obedient to Christ" (2 Cor. 10:5 NIV) and to "be self-controlled and alert. Your enemy the devil prowls around like a roaring lion looking for someone to devour" (1 Peter 5:8). As the regressionist and client throw themselves into the pit of hypnotic delusion, they confidently expect the Holy Spirit to safely guide them through because they "prayed." In violating God's commands, we can't then turn around and expect that He will protect us when we are practicing hollow and deceptive philosophies. C. S. Lewis commented:

> There are, no doubt, passages in the New Testament which may seem at first sight to promise an invariable granting of our prayers. But that cannot be what they really mean. For in the very heart of the story we meet a glaring instance to the contrary. In Gethsemane the holiest of all petitioners prayed three

times that a certain cup might pass from Him. It did not. After that the idea that prayer is recommended to us as a sort of infallible gimmick may be dismissed.[5]

"What's the biblical standard for accepting an accusation against another person?"

What about Steve's claim that he doesn't need to discover the truth of an accusation? This is an assumption that I've encountered with every regressionist I've talked to so far. You see, they insist that they aren't detectives and therefore don't need to investigate criminal allegations. This certainly sounds reasonable. But is Scripture's standard for accepting accusations really what they are teaching? Are we just supposed to pray and "take it on faith" that whatever fantasies our mind develops are from God? Is it really not the Christian's job "to try to find out the truth" when someone is accused of rape and murder? Are we to sit in judgment against entire families and refuse to involve them or allow any evidence that would defend their innocence?

More than anyone else in history, Jesus Christ knows what it is to be falsely accused. His persecutors also held to the same standard for "justice." Washing their hands, they were sure that it was someone else's job. Again we turn to Scripture, and in doing so we discover that God's perspective is radically different and holds us to a higher standard regarding accusations. In Deuteronomy 19:15, 18–19, God declared:

> One witness is not enough to convict a man accused of any crime or offense he may have committed. A matter must be established by the testimony of two or three witnesses. . . . The judges must make a thorough investigation, and if the witness proves to be a liar, giving false testimony against his brother, then do to him as he intended to do to his brother. You must purge the evil from among you. (NIV)

This is the same passage that Christ reaffirmed in Matthew 18:16: "Take one or two others along, so that 'every matter may be established by the testimony of two or three witnesses'" (NIV).

God's standard for protecting against false accusations becomes even more imperative when the person is making them based on hypnotic fantasies he has experienced during the course of self- or therapist-induced trance. Remember, a hypnotic fantasy of a traumatic event is in no way evidence that any crime has taken place and is, in fact, actually less likely to be accurate or real. Without solid, external evidence, there is no way for a treating therapist to know its authenticity. We have a duty to discover the truth, and we must withhold judgment until we have conclusive evidence.

Notice that God's standard does not dismiss the need to investigate even if a person does not have a history of exaggeration or of reporting being told something "that God wouldn't say." Satan himself used the very words of God when he was tempting Christ in the wilderness. One would think that he's bright enough to introduce seductive fantasies that are tailor-made to fit the client's and therapist's prior expectations. We should expect that a satanic deception will sound just like something God would have said. The more closely a lie resembles the truth, the more powerful is its ability to deceive.

The Scriptures Speak

Here's what we've discovered so far: Regression is not a biblical concept or practice. There is no difference between regular hypnosis and the brand that Christian regressionists call "Holy Spirit guidance." Prayer is not a magical incantation that will protect us from foolish choices. And finally, we have a duty to discover the truth of an accusation and are not allowed the option to stand in judgment against someone who is accused based on hypnotic fantasies. So far, we know the Bible doesn't support the claims of regressionists. What else can we learn from Scripture on these issues?

"What is the nature of our adversary?"

The Bible teaches that Satan has devoted himself to opposing God and His creation. Jesus describes him as a thief who comes only to "steal, and kill, and to destroy" (John 10:10). In addition to being our adversary he also seeks to accuse us. In fact, the name "Satan" comes from a Hebrew word meaning "adversary" and/or "accuser." Scripture points us to his accusing nature in Revelation 12:10 where he is described as the "accuser of our brethren" (see also Zech. 3:1). He is a master of deception, described as a "father of lies" who is able to masquerade as "an angel of light" and produce "counterfeit miracles, signs, and wonders" in order to deceive others (John 8:44, 2 Cor. 11:14, and 2 Thess. 2:9–10).

Interestingly, when I was practicing regressionism, I was living within a powerful contradiction. While having believed in mythical legions of multigenerational satanists, I had simultaneously ignored the real nature of Satan which is taught in Scripture, including his advanced ability to accuse and deceive. Is it possible that Satan, in a macabre twist to Paul's words in 1 Corinthians 9:22, is able to be "all things to all men," accommodating whatever belief system a person has? For the feminists under hypnosis, is this master of deception and accusation able to provide fantasies of incestuous white patriarchs? Does he satisfy the New Agers' desires to embrace colorful past lives or almond-eyed space aliens? Could it be that as Christians have opened themselves up to regression techniques, an "angel of light" has responded to their invitation and led them to a horrifying new gospel? "The Spirit clearly says that in later times some will abandon the faith and follow deceiving spirits and things taught by demons" (1 Tim. 4:1 NIV). Could it be that in these later times this prophecy is being fulfilled? When I was practicing regressionism, I sat with my hypnotized clients, pen in hand, taking down every detail of their hypnotic images. I was truly believing that what they were seeing could only be real. But what if the images were otherwise? John gave us a clear warning: "Dear friends, do not believe every spirit, but test the spirits to see whether they are from God, because many false prophets have gone out into the world" (1 John 4:1). What if Satan doesn't need legions of multigenerational satanists? What if he already has thousands of zealous Christian regressionists who are eagerly responding to every fantasy suggested by hypnotized clients?

This certainly was the case for over three hundred years of witch-hunting, in which thousands of Christians were tortured and murdered because Christian oppressors believed they were following the leading of God. Today, as in those days, we find no evidence of multigenerational satanists. But there is clear evidence that the regressionists, often in the name of Christ, are bringing about false accusations, the destruction of individual lives, and the devastation of thousands of families.

That said, I want to explain something very clearly. It is not my intention to suggest that everyone involved in the regression movement is demon-possessed or oppressed. As a Christian and a psychologist, I'm trying to make sense out of what is going on within this movement. What I do know is this: Scripture is clear that Satan has an adverse effect on believers when we follow his leading. In working with hundreds of individuals and families in the False Memory Crisis I've discovered that the divorces, suicides, raging emotions, selfishness, and destroyed families that result from regression therapy are consistent with his goals.

Another precaution: We don't want to turn Satan into a scapegoat—"The devil made me do it!"—thus relieving ourselves from personal responsibility for our own choices. Satan is a powerful created being who is in rebellion against God and seeks to destroy His creation. But his power is limited and his influence does not exclude us from responsibility for our own choices. He cannot dominate us except by our own consent and believers will not be tempted beyond their power of resistance (1 Cor. 10:13). We have the protection of the Holy Spirit through the armor of God (Eph. 6:11-18), as long as we choose to use it, peace through His indwelling, and the revelation of truth through our relationship with Christ and Scripture. All of these gifts are given to us as effective countermeasures against Satan's influence.

Deception in Christian Garb

Jon Trott, from *Cornerstone* magazine, comments:

Christians must be on the forefront of reaffirming the importance of critical thought. We should be looking for ways to guard our brother or sister against being abused by stories without any evidence. And if we're the gullible ones, we must be willing to admit our need![6]

He quotes Bill Backus:

I have clients tell me, "I went up to the altar for prayer and the elder who prayed with me, laid hands on me, said 'I think you've been abused.'" And the person isn't adequately taught by the church how to evaluate that. The church shouldn't be doing that in the first place. But at least there ought to be teaching on how to skeptically evaluate other people's supposedly Spirit-given information.[7]

The issue of regressionism actually speaks to a much broader crisis within the Church today. We've gradually allowed our beliefs to be defined by novel experiences rather than drawing from a biblical perspective. First we experience an exciting, "miraculous" event, like recovered memories, then we go back to Scripture and make it say what we want it to. Theology that is defined by experience introduces tremendous dangers, especially when the experience is in contradiction to the Word of God. Is it any wonder that evil in the latter days will be known by its "counterfeit miracles, signs and wonders, and in every sort of evil that deceives those who are perishing" (2 Thess. 2:9–10 NIV). In addition we know that "the time will come when men will not put up with sound doctrine. Instead, to suit their own desires, they will gather around them a great number of teachers to say what their itching ears want to hear. They will turn their ears away from the truth and turn aside to myths" (2 Tim. 4:3–4 NIV).

Is it possible that thousands of Christian regressionists have abandoned the standard of revealed truth and have instead come to accept fraudulent "miracles" as real? This much we know for sure, the supernatural events we experience must be in accordance with Scripture and not the latest therapeutic craze. The Bible has rightly warned us, "See to it that no one takes you captive through hollow and deceptive philosophy . . ." (Col. 2:8 NIV).

We can expect that deception will come, especially from within our own ranks in the Church. Scripture has important insights concerning false teachings in the latter days, noting that leaders will come to us in sheep's clothing but inwardly be as ferocious as wolves (Matt. 7:15). They will arise within the Christian community and secretly introduce destructive heresies, based on stories they have made up (2 Peter 2:1). They are described as false apostles and deceitful workmen who are excellent in following their master, who masquerades as an angel of light (2 Cor. 11:13). They will worm their way into homes and gain control over weak-willed women, who are loaded down with sins and swayed by all kinds of evil desires. These false teachers will be always learning but never able to acknowledge the truth (2 Tim. 3:5–7). "Such a person goes into great detail about what he has seen, and his unspiritual mind puffs him up with idle notions" (Col. 2:18 NIV).

In turn, followers of false teachers will learn their shameful ways and bring the truth into disrepute (2 Peter 2:2). They will be lovers of themselves, boastful, disobedient to their parents, ungrateful, without love, unforgiving, slanderous, without self-control, brutal, conceited, and having a form of godliness but denying its power (2 Tim. 3:1–5). They will even rebel against their parents and have them put to death (Matt. 10:21).

Could it be that, from two thousand years ago, the Bible has described the movement of our times? Regression leaders, dressed in Christian garb and "God talk," have arisen within the body of Christ and introduced a dangerous new gospel. In the name of psychotherapy, they have enticed vulnerable women into believing that they are the victims of abuse, based on scary urban myths, "symptoms lists," and hypnotic inductions. With deep conviction and sincerity, regressionists teach their followers that they must spend years searching into the past using special mind-altering techniques, and they must accept their hypnotic fantasies as absolute truth. They are always finding newly recovered memories but are never able to acknowledge the truth that their doctrines and practices fly in the face of science and Scripture. I always believed that verses concerning deception in the end times would be fulfilled. What I never suspected was that thousands of Christians, myself included, would play such an active role in bringing them about.

Many in the body of Christ have openly embraced the deception of regressionism and satanic panic. We must face the painful truth of our deception and work to allow the Holy Spirit to undo the destruction that the enemy has brought into the homes and hearts of so many. Father Cornelius Loos actively opposed the witch-hunts of his time, and as a result he was horribly tortured. From four hundred years ago, his words call out to us today: "One can but exclaim, O Christian Religion, how long shalt thou be vexed with this direst of superstitions? and cry aloud, O Christian Commonwealth, how long in thee shall the life of the innocent be imperiled?"[8]

Awakening the Sleeping Giant: A Call to the Church

Christ wants me to see, to see far and to see truly. To get
that kind of vision requires avoidance of hypocrisies and group
prejudice which distort the vision and make men imagine they
see what is not really there.
JOHN FOSTER DULLES

"Michael" was the pastor of a large fellowship, which had its own counseling center with several therapists who were strong regression activists. In a seminar sponsored by his church, I described the dangers of regression therapy and the need to address this crisis. I noticed that Michael hadn't been in attendance. Later I spoke with him, curious as to why he had gone to the expense and effort to bring me out to speak, yet hadn't taken the time to listen in. He explained,

"The issue of recovered memories is a psychological debate. It's up to the professionals to figure it out. It's simply not my job."

Unfortunately this is a common attitude that I've encountered with many Christians, who assume the "experts" have a better handle on this issue and it's best left up to them. Through the media and the courts our nation is beginning to come to terms with the False Memory Crisis. But within the Church there is still a deep slumber, as we continue to accept the claims of recovered memories with little questioning. However the alarm has sounded, as we too are forced to address the crisis in our midst. Thousands of families have stepped forward to identify themselves as the true victims—victims of a movement that has spun out of control. Are all the families perpetrators, satanists, simply in "denial"? Or is there something to their claims of false accusation? A growing number of retractors are asserting that they have been the victims of abusive and suggestive therapies, in which they came to believe in horrific fantasies. Are all these people simply denying the reality of their abuse? Proverbs 18:17 warns us, "The first to present his case seems right, till another comes forward and questions him" (NIV). Could it be that we have failed to allow for the other side of this tragedy a voice of defense? The business of truth is central to the mission of the church—we should be at the forefront challenging regressionists' claims and reaching out to those who have been harmed in this movement. Now, more than ever, is the time for us to "Stop judging by mere appearances, and make a right judgment" (John 7:24 NIV).

A Quest for Truth

It is never safe to attribute a man's imaginations too
directly to his experience.
C. S. LEWIS[9]

Scripture is clear in commanding us to question doctrines that are not consistent with God's revealed truth. The Church is in a position to bring powerful healing in the False Memory Crisis. To accomplish this we need an uncompromising commitment to Christ's truth—an unwavering seeking, testing, and speaking of truth.

Seek the Truth

Let's be honest. We're preprogrammed for deception. We love exotic tales, to have our ears tickled by exciting stories. The notion that we can regress back into the womb, that there are thousands of murdering satanists out there, that's novel and exciting! In comparison, the possibility that these ideas are the product of hypnotic techniques, mental disorders, or urban rumors is boring. "The coming of the lawless one will be in accordance with the work of Satan displayed in all kinds of counterfeit miracles, signs and wonders, and in every sort of evil that deceives those who are perishing. They perish because they refused to love the truth and so be saved." (2 Thess. 2:9-10 NIV). One of the things we learn from Paul's teaching is that believers will be fooled by counterfeit miracles because we refused to love the truth. In our learning to discern we must first become lovers of the truth. We have to desire it more than our natural desire for the fantastic, our busy schedules, or reluctance to avoid offending someone (see Gen. 6:5 and 8:21).

You see, it's easier and more comfortable to believe an accusation, to reach a conclusion, than it is to prove it. The process of investigating a claim as described in Deuteronomy 19:15-19 is time-consuming and creates discomfort when the accuser is demanding that you accept the theories and techniques of regressionism as true. But Scripture is very clear in asserting that we aren't given the option to simply take accusations against another without investigating the matter. Christ tells us, "Seek, and you will find; knock, and it will be opened to you" (Matt. 7:7 NIV). The good news is that Jesus assures us that if we seek the truth, we will find it, but to do so we have to actually get up off the couch and make the effort to knock on doors. It means hearing both sides—"How could the theory of regressionism be false?" "How would you know someone's claim of abuse is a fantasy created in her mind?" There will be those who forbid you to seek, refuse your questions, shame you for requiring evidence. A caring skepticism is dangerous to those who aren't grounded in biblical truth.

Are you ready to love the truth? To desire it more than being accepted? To move out of your comfort zone in your search? Be forewarned, to question this movement means you run the risk of being accused as well. The seeker of truth is pulled into the line of fire for those who would oppose it.

"Knowledge is two-fold, and consists not only in an affirmation of what is true, but in the negation of that which is false"
CHARLES CALEB COLTON, 1825.

Test the Truth

The next step in evaluating regressionism is to test the claims and teachings that we come across. C. S. Lewis noted, "We should never ask of anything 'Is it real?,' for everything is real. The proper question is 'A real what?' e.g., a real snake or real delirium tremens?"[10] Hypnotic images of incest, ritual abuse, space alien abductions, and prior lives feel real, have intense emotions and detail. It's not a question of whether these images are real—they *are* real to the person having them. The question is, as C. S. Lewis said, the images are a real *what*? A true memory or a therapist-induced fantasy? My pastor, Tom Copps, regularly reminds me of an important principle, "Subjective revelation must always yield to objective revelation." *Subjective revelation* is what happens when someone claims to have had a special word or teaching from the Lord, whereas *objective revelation* is revealed in the Bible. Most Christians, myself included, can point to a time in our lives in which we've felt a direct leading from God concerning some matter. But subjective experience must always correlate with the objective standard that is provided to us in Scripture. Just because someone claims "the Holy Spirit revealed this to me" doesn't end the matter of verification. In fact, it begins it. Christians are commanded to have "nothing to do with godless myths and old wives' tales" (1 Tim. 4:7 NIV). John's warning is very clear, "Beloved, do not believe every spirit, but test the spirits, whether they are of God; because many false prophets have gone out into the world" (1 John 4:1). If a teaching or theory is God's truth, it will hold up under closer examination. Our ability to question is one of the most important tools we have in combating deception and we must be prepared to ask tough ones.

In this chapter we've examined questions that Christians need to ask (i.e., "Is this in keeping with Scripture?"). Let me suggest another important one: "What's the fruit of this work?" In Matthew 7:15–17, Jesus warns us:

> Beware of false prophets, who come to you in sheep's clothing, but inwardly they are ravenous wolves. You will know them by their fruits. Do men gather grapes from thornbushes or figs from thistles? Even so, every good tree bears good fruit, but a bad tree bears bad fruit.

What exactly does this "good fruit" that Jesus spoke of look like? Galatians 5:22-23 reveals, "But the fruit of the Spirit is love, joy, peace, longsuffering, kindness, goodness, faithfulness, gentleness, self-control." The life of a believer also gives us clues as to whether God is at work within him or her: "For God has not given us a spirit of fear, but of power and of love and of a sound mind" (2 Tim. 1:7). Galatians 6:7–8 warns us, "Do not be deceived, God is not mocked; for whatever a man sows, that will he also reap. For he who sows to his flesh will of the flesh reap corruption, but he who sows to the Spirit will of the Spirit reap everlasting life." In 2 Timothy 3:1–5 we're told:

> But know this, that in the last days perilous times will come: For men will be lovers of themselves, lovers of money, boasters, proud, blasphemers, disobedient to parents, unthankful, unholy, unloving, unforgiving, slanderers, without self-control, brutal, despisers of good, traitors, headstrong, haughty, lovers of pleasure rather than lovers of God, having a form of godliness but denying its power. And from such people turn away!

When I was doing regression therapies I watched reasonably healthy people degenerate into psychotic, out-of-control personalities. These new creations were raging, constantly suicidal, selfish, and demanding. Eventually they were unable to work, to parent, to survive outside of my office. Divorces followed and patients ruthlessly cut off anyone who questioned their hypnotic images or their endless accusations. Despite their worsening condition, they embraced and nurtured their status as "victim." Their hatred toward their parents expanded into grotesque proportions as they realized within themselves the apostle Paul's ominous warning, "'Honor your father and mother,' which is the first commandment with a promise: 'that it may be well with you and you may enjoy long life on the earth'" (Eph. 6:2–3). Clearly things were not going well with regression believers.

I watched entire churches get caught up in the hysteria, creating "safe houses" to hide self-described SRA survivors. I watched churches and Christian colleges get ripped apart by the accusations that regression believers generated. In one case an entire missionary team was dismantled because one of the members went into regression therapy while on leave, only to rejoin the team and wreak havoc upon the others. Scripture calls out to us, "You ran well. Who hindered you from obeying the truth? This persuasion does not come from Him who calls you" (Gal. 5:7–8). Is this the Holy Spirit at work in believers' lives? Does regressionism really bear the fruit we would expect? This much is clear for me: In all my work promoting recovered memories and later in critiquing this movement, I have yet to meet a single person whose life and family were actually better after she experienced her hypnotic fantasies.

Speaking the Truth

Not only do we have a duty to search and test the truth, the Bible calls us to proclaim it as well, to take a stand against those who would deceive others.

> We should no longer be children, tossed to and fro and carried about with every wind of doctrine, by the trickery of men, in the cunning craftiness of deceitful plotting, but, speaking the truth in love, may grow up in all things into Him who is the head—Christ. (Eph. 4:14–15)

It is not enough that we simply recognize the False Memory Crisis is happening around and within us. We must act according to Proverbs 24:11–12:

> Deliver those who are drawn toward death,
> And hold back those stumbling to the slaughter.
> If you say, "Surely we did not know this,"
> Does not He who weighs the hearts consider it?
> He who keeps your soul, does He not know it?
> And will He not render to each man according to his deeds?

As we come to recognize the reality of the False Memory Crisis, we are faced with the challenge of becoming proactive in dealing with regression promoters, "true believers," accused families, retractors, and those who have been truly abused.

A) Regression Leaders

"If we find a man giving pleasure it is for us to prove (if we criticize him) that his action is wrong. But if we find a man inflicting pain it is for him to prove that his action is right. If he cannot, he is a wicked man."

C. S. LEWIS, *GOD IN THE DOCK*, 1947[11]

The Church needs to hold regressionists accountable for what they are teaching and practicing within the Christian community—either it is true or it is something else—on the explosive issue of regressionism there is an imperative need to determine which. Within the Body of Christ we know that true doctrine and practice matters. If someone is promoting a doctrine that is contrary to the Bible, we have a duty to correct that person in love. But John Locke points out, "It is one thing to show a man that he is in error, and another to put him in possession of truth." If a regressionist refuses to listen to reason and truth, the Church is left in an uncomfortable, but necessary, position of dealing with them. In Titus 3:10, Paul tells us: "Warn a divisive person once, and then warn him a second time. After that, have nothing to do with him." (NIV). In 2 John 1:9–11 we are told;

> Anyone who runs ahead and does not continue in the teaching of Christ does not have God; whoever continues in the teaching has both the Father and the Son. If anyone comes to you and does not bring this teaching, do not take him into your house or welcome him. Anyone who welcomes him shares in his wicked work. (NIV)

We also need to keep in mind that many therapists are simply caught in the middle. They aren't actively promoting repressed memories, but they have clients who are coming to them hurting and claiming to have recovered traumatic images from the past. These therapists are understandably uncertain of how to proceed. Nonetheless, they have a duty to communicate truth to their clients—not simply to say the things that will please. With regard to recovered memories of abuse, there's simply no way that a therapist or client can determine the validity of the images apart from solid, external corroborating evidence. Furthermore, we know that if those images were recovered in the context of previous regression therapy and its techniques, the resulting fantasies are less likely to reflect real events. With an unflinching commitment to the truth, this needs to be communicated to clients by their therapists.

B) Regression Believers

Regarding the "true believers" caught up in the movement. How does the Church respond to their claims? The world's system tells us that we aren't to question them. But Scripture gives us a radically different standard and command. The challenge for the Church is to develop an approach that listens to their claims with a caring skepticism and allows for the accused to have a fair hearing as well.

On another point, regression believers are the most miserable people I know. Their hypnotic fantasies have led them into an ever-descending litany of despair, self-abuse, fear and loneliness. Having abandoned their loved ones they are left with their "therapeutic" families, which only feeds their downward spiral. The truth of violating Ephesians 6:2–3, ". . . 'that it may go well with you and that you may enjoy long life on the earth,'" (NIV) is borne out within their lives. While there is a growing number of resources that can help them move out of regressionism—many simply refuse to hear any evidence that would contradict their fantasies. C. S. Lewis notes, "I willingly believe that the damned are, in one sense, successful, rebels to the end; that the doors of hell are locked on the inside."[12] The fact that regression believers have locked themselves inside their own living hell only makes their agony all the more senseless. The Church faces the challenge of how to reach out to them with healing and truth yet at the same time hold them accountable for choices they have made.

C) The Accused

As noted earlier, more than any person in history, Jesus Christ knows what it is to be falsely accused. His killers abandoned the search for truth because His guilty verdict was politically popular and expedient. Sometimes I've wondered, if I was there would I have denied Him as well? Would I have opposed the thousands to defend His right to a fair trial? You and I are afforded the opportunity to answer those questions every day, in the here and now. Within our churches and society there are thousands of families that have been destroyed by accusations based on fantasies and fraudulent therapies. Regressionism has been devastating for them. Not only have they lost their daughters and sons to this movement—in turn their lives have been turned upside down. Will we stand in the face of a public hysteria that demands a guilty verdict? Will we call out for the right to a fair hearing? Does truth matter?

We must find ways to reach out to the accused and minister to them in their agony. One way the Church can assist is allowing the accused to have a voice in the process, providing a "middle ground" in which the accused can meet with their accuser. My fervent hope is that churches will step up to the challenges of the False Memory Crisis and develop an alternative that allows for both sides to make their case.

D) Retractors

As the False Memory Crisis comes to light an increasing number of women and men are stepping out of their therapies bewildered, angry, and ashamed. Most of the retractors I've worked with were Christians when they began their descent into regressionism. They had Christian therapists that they trusted and "godtalk" that made the theories and techniques sound scientific and biblical. After having escaped from their therapeutic tortures, they came away with their faith in pieces and unsure of what aspects of their Christian teaching they could trust anymore. Many dropped out of church all together—the pain was simply too much to bear. They carry deep shame and regret over their choices, accusations, years lost. They are furious about their mind-rape, in many instances sponsored by the church leaders they trusted most.

The Church faces the challenge of reaching out to these regression survivors. How do we minister to their needs? How do we help them be restored to the Christian faith? Can we play a role in helping them to reconcile with their families—to know forgiveness and true healing? This next stage in the False Memory Crisis presents some of the most difficult challenges. Yet it also affords an opportunity for the Church to minister and help reconcile retractors back to God and their families.

E) Real Victims of Abuse

In my counseling practice I continue to work with victims of abuse. Recently I've had an increasing number of clients with free-standing memories wondering if they might have false memories. It's ironic that a movement intended to heal victims has resulted in real victims being hurt and discounted. In dealing with those who have been affected by regressionism, situations arise that are remarkably similar to Jesus' portrayal of a harvest gone wrong, where weeds were sown by an enemy in the midst of good wheat. Many cases of abuse are all too real. But what about the "forgotten memories" from decades or centuries ago that emerge under the guidance of a regressionist? The "father of lies" and "accuser of the brethren" has created a powerful double bind. By pulling at the weeds sown by regressionists we risk harming true abuse victims. And it doesn't take a genius to figure out that the next strategy regression believers have taken is to assert that their memories have "always" been remembered, whereby they mean their unconscious or cells in their body have always held the event (what they won't tell you is that it was only recently this information was released into conscious awareness). In a similar vein I've recently had discussions with regressionists who have dropped the word "regression" and "repression" from their vocabulary. Instead they speak of clients who "dissociated" their traumas or experienced psychogenic amnesia. They desperately believe that by renaming their theories and techniques they will somehow be exempted from all the findings we've discussed in this book.

If all of this feels confusing, understand that they intend it to be. The more effectively regression believers can camouflage themselves amongst the real thing, use distracting labels and "victim speak" the tougher it is to weed them out. It is imperative that we find discernment in claims of abuse, so that true victims are not neglected and innocent lives are not destroyed through false accusations (Prov. 17:15). We can accomplish this by applying ourselves to a Biblical course of action and develop a caring skepticism with regard to recovered memory claims. It's about finding balance. Regressionism's claims, with all its potential for personal devastation, must be handled with an uncompromising commitment to the Truth. You see, it's easy for us as Christians to write off space alien abductions and past life traumas, because they're not part of our belief system. But what if someone has a delusion that fits into our belief system? If Satan, the "father of lies," wanted to deceive a Christian, would he appear to him as a space alien or an Angel of Light? Scripture and church history give us the answer.

This much I do know, in the end we will all stand before the Author of Truth, who is passionately committed to justice. In that moment He'll ask us if we defended Him against false accusations, did we stand for Him when others cried out for conviction? Some no doubt will ask, "Lord, when were You falsely accused? I wasn't part of the crowd that stood against You and cried out for Your conviction. I lived in the twentieth century, long after the fact." From Matthew 25:40 we learn the Lord's response: "I tell you the truth, whatever you did for one of the least of these brothers of mine, you did for me" (NIV). In that moment some will discover that they spent a lifetime looking the other way, seeking out their own safety, concluding that some matters were simply too complicated. Others will have stepped into controversies, fought for justice—the right to a fair hearing, risked their own for others. In the end each of us makes our choices, day-to-day decisions that either take Christ down off the Cross or put Him back upon it.

Points to Remember

In coming to terms with the spiritual dimension of the False Memory Crisis, we discover:

✓ Regressionism is not in harmony with Scripture and fails the test of General and Special Revelation.

✓ The use of "Holy Spirit Guides" in memory recovery has no biblical precedent or support and is simply a renaming of common hypnotic techniques. This is an example of "god-talk" that is commonly used by regressionists to promote their theories and techniques as valid.

✓ The Bible does *not* teach us that prayer will automatically protect us from foolish choices or violating God's principles.

✓ The practices of regressionism are in direct contradiction to biblical standards for accepting an accusation against another person.

✓ The fruit of the recovered memory movement is consistent with the results that we would expect from the "father of lies" and "accuser of the brethren." It is also in keeping with the deception that is prophesied to occur in latter days.

✓ In responding to the False Memory Crisis, Christians have a duty to seek the truth, test the truth, and speak the truth.

Facing the Storm

*Nothing in all the world is more dangerous than sincere ignorance
and conscientious stupidity.*

MARTIN LUTHER KING, JR., STRENGTH TO LOVE, 1963

In 1718 Bishop Francis Hutchinson wrote about the witch-hunts of his day. "If the same notions were to prevail again (and super-stition is never far off), no man's life would be safe in his own house, for the fantastic doctrines that support the vulgar opinions of witchcraft rob us of all the defenses that God and Nature have placed for our security against false accusations. For in other cases, when wicked or mistaken people charge us with crimes of which we are not guilty, we clear ourselves by showing that at that time we were at home, or in some other place, about our honest busi-ness. But in prosecutions for witchcraft, that most natural and just defense is a mere jest; for if any wicked person affirms, or any crackbrained girl imagines, or any lying spirit makes her believe, that she sees any old woman, or other person pursuing her in her visions, the defenders of the vulgar witchcraft tack an imaginary, unproved compact to the deposition, and hang the accused parties for things that they were doing when they were, perhaps, asleep upon their beds, or saying their prayers, or, perhaps, in the accuser's own possession, with double irons upon them. But such fantastic notions are so far from raising their sickly visions into legal evidence, that they are grounded upon the very dregs of pagan and popish superstitions, and leave the lives of innocent men naked without defense against them."[1]

The Resurrection of the Hunt

The rebirth of the witch-hunts today represents what is arguably the single greatest threat to our society and its members. Every person, every priest and pastor, every parent with a savings account, every public figure, every Christian believer whose faith is inconvenient to others, every school teacher, anyone can be the target of the hunt and its fantasy accusations. Think about this for a moment, whether it was yesterday or decades ago, every child you have ever known, ever had the slightest contact with, even your very own children—can have fantasies created within them that will target you as an abuser. There is no charge that is too fantastic, too unbelievable that those around you will not assume your guilt, after all they don't want you perpetrating on their children! With eyes ablaze with righteous zeal, your accusers will seek to destroy you as their service to God and man.

So tell me, how would you defend yourself from something alleged to have happened decades ago? Stop for a moment, really answer this question. How would you prove that you didn't rape a little girl thirty years ago? Someone tells your entire church that decades in the past you wore black robes and committed unspeakable crimes in the name of Satan. She affirms this by saying it was the Holy Spirit that revealed these things to her. Remember, "if any wicked person affirms, or any crackbrained girl imagines, or any lying spirit makes her believe" that you have committed these crimes, how will you prove her false? What evidence could you produce that proves you didn't do this.

I'm waiting.

It's so easy to throw stones. It's so easy to assume that those who are accused have done something wrong! But once you've been pulled into hysteria's grip, been accused, been tainted—then it's too late to exclaim "Now I understand!" You've joined the ranks of "them" and anything you say or do can be easily explained away as the protests of a perpetrator. The genius of hysteria is that, once the label is applied (witch, communist, abuser, satanist) there is no defense, no evidence that cannot be explained away. Pamela Freyd, director of the FMS Foundation, notes:

> An accusation of sexual abuse creates a stigma that probably lasts forever. In November of 1995, *Dateline* asked 502 adults, "If someone has been charged and acquitted in a child abuse case, would you still be suspicious of them?" Poll results showed . . . an overwhelming majority, 77% said yes, they would still be suspicious, even if the suspect was cleared. When a therapist makes a diagnosis of incest based on a "recovered memory," he or she gives a lifetime sentence to the accused.[2]

In a moment your life as you have known it will have ended. Years of reputation, ministry, career are over. Lifetime family relationships will be terminated—you will lose your children, grandchildren, maybe even your spouse. You might be convicted and sentenced to prison, lose your home, your lifetime savings. You will enter into a hell shared today by hundreds of thousands of family members and join the ranks of countless falsely accused from across the centuries. In that moment you will know the sweeping devastation of the False Memory Crisis.

Is there hope? I'm glad you asked.

Justice Comes Calling

"There is nothing concealed that will not be disclosed, or hidden that will not be made known. What you have said in the dark will be heard in the daylight, and what you have whispered in the ear in the inner rooms will be proclaimed from the housetops."

JESUS CHRIST, LUKE 12:2–3 (NIV)

Eileen Franklin says that she was looking into the eyes of her young daughter when she got her first "flashback." She claims she suddenly remembered twenty years earlier her father, George Franklin, raising a rock over her playmate, Susan Nason's, head. This playmate had in fact been murdered two decades prior and the crime had remained unsolved. What ensued was one of the most sensational trials of the regression movement and the first conviction brought about based on a recovered memory. On her testimony alone, without any other corroborating evidence, her father was convicted and sentenced to a lifetime in jail. As his life faded into a lonely, black nightmare, Eileen went on to become a popular star of the recovered memory movement—she wrote a couple books, got on the national speaking circuit and even had a TV movie done on her "ordeal." That was several years ago.

I'm looking at this morning's newspaper. George Franklin is being released from prison today, an innocent man who had been falsely imprisoned. It was only after the trial was completed that law enforcement got the compete story. The details that Eileen had "recovered" were presented to the jury as "inside" information that only an actual witness to the murder could have known. Turns out those details were available to anyone who had read the newspapers from twenty years ago, which a witness later said Eileen had done before the trial. Earlier Eileen had claimed that her father had also committed a second murder. But recent DNA tests have cleared George of any possible involvement. Eileen had testified that she hadn't been hypnotized, that the "memories" were spontaneous. Her sister testified last month that both she and Eileen had been hypnotized by a therapist before the trial had begun. An innocent man, whose life was destroyed at the height of regression hysteria, is able to live once more as a free man. His attorney laments that George lost six years of his life because of "voodoo therapy."

After enjoying years of popularity, regressionism has recently fallen upon hard times. Today's headlines tell the story:

Arizona Daily Star
Restored-memory Suits Going Against Therapists

A psychiatrist has been ordered to pay $350,000 for telling a woman's family he believed her parents sexually abused her 40 years ago....[3]

Knoxville News Sentinel
Sexual Abuse Suit Dismissed

An $8 million lawsuit brought by two daughters of an Oak Ridge physicist has been dismissed. The daughters alleged that the father abused them "on many and frequent occasions ... during their childhood," and they repressed the memories....[4]

Newsday
Judge Kills Nun's Sex Suit

A $3.75 million civil suit filed by a Long Island nun who said she was sexually abused by her mother superior more than 25 years ago have been dismissed because the statute of limitations for bringing the charge has expired.... "New York law does not recognize psychological trauma or repression as justification for avoiding the statute of limitations."[5]

Grand Rapids Press
Accused Michigan Father
Acquitted in Allegan County Trial

After experiencing flashbacks and repressed memories, a daughter tried to sue her father. After deliberating less than an hour and a half the jury brought back a "not guilty" decision. One juror noted, "I think if you're going to accuse someone, you have to have more evidence than the memories. It just seemed like such a weak case to me. I was a little surprised it made it to court." Her parents share, "I know that we love her—an unconditional love. We'd take her back any day; take her back any time."[6]

The San Diego Union-Tribune
Father Settles for $2.5 Million in Rape Case

A former Navy man falsely accused of raping his daughter would get $2.5 million under a tentative settlement of his lawsuit against government agencies and individuals. . . . The pact would end a five year tragedy and official bungling.[7]

Associated Press
Psychiatrist and Hospital Found Negligent

A jury awards more than $272,000 to a former client for being improperly diagnosed and treated when she was encouraged to believe in nonexistent events and disregarded information that contradicted the allegations of abuse. A separate lawsuit is still pending against prosecutors, social workers, police detectives and child advocacy attorneys. . . .[8]

Dallas Morning News
Jury Finds Psychiatrist Liable in Slander Suit

A Dallas County jury awarded $350,000 to a couple for slander by a psychiatrist who asserted to their daughter and grandchildren that they were perpetrators. The daughter reconciled to the parents and the lawsuit followed. They hope that the verdict will prevent this kind of thing from happening to other families and that the verdict "has the effect of making psychiatrists and others in the mental health field think very carefully before making statements that are not true about someone else."[9]

Houston Chronicle
Suit Hits Satanism Memories

A $50 million dollar lawsuit has been filed by a former patient for conspiracy, negligence and fraud related to 3 1/2 years of therapy that cost her insurance company more than $3 million dollars. She was convinced by doctors that her depression and anxiety were indications of repressed memories of childhood abuse. She came to believe she was a member of a satanic cult and had practiced human sacrifices.[10]

The Arizona Daily Star
Center Accused of Planting False Memories

The families of 5 patients at a Christian counseling center in Scottsdale, Arizona, filed complaints with the Arizona Board of Behavioral Health Examiners. . . .[11]

The Arizona Republic
Counselor Hit with Another Suit

Another lawsuit has been filed against an embattled Scottsdale counselor and others accused of planting "false memories" of child sexual abuse and Satanism during therapy.[12]

Minneapolis-St. Paul Star Tribune
Jurors Award $2.6 Million for False Memories

A former client successfully sued her psychiatrist for more than $2.6 million for being mis diagnosed as "MPD" and being told she must have been sexually abused. In addition, she was awarded $461,000 for future damages and her husband was awarded $210,000 for loss of partnership. The former client shares, "I'm really very glad. It's been a long seven years"[13]

Arizona Daily Star, Associated Press
Therapists Planted False Childhood Memories in Woman, Jury Rules

Napa, Calif. (AP) Two therapists destroyed a father's life by implanting false memories of child abuse in his daughter's mind, a jury ruled yesterday. The jurors awarded the father $500,000 in damages.[14]

The National Law Journal
"False" Memory, Big Award

Juries are penalizing therapists who evoke "repressed" memories of abuse. . . .[15]

The Party Is Over

As the witch-hunts progressed, Friedrich von Spee wrote:

Thus eventually those who at first clamored most loudly to feed the flames are themselves involved, for they rashly failed to see that their turn too would come. Thus Heaven justly punishes those who with their pestilent tongues created so many witches and sent so many innocent to the stake. . . . Now many of the wiser and more learned judges are opening their eyes to this enormity, and proceed more slowly and cautiously.[16]

Finally, the same caution is being taken by our law-enforcement offices.

Behind the closed doors of the regressionist's office, unproved theories were espoused and lives were destroyed. Sincerely believing that what they were doing was right, regressionists continued their dangerous practices, certain that rules of confidentiality would protect them. But this thinking has been a prelude to the final revelation described in Luke 12:2 3: "For there is nothing covered that will not be revealed, nor hidden that will not be known. Therefore whatever you have spoken in the dark will be heard in the light, and what you have spoken in the ear in inner rooms will be proclaimed on the housetops." In our research with retractors, we found that 63 percent of retractors had initiated legal action against their therapists.[17] Ironically, it isn't the pedophiles, the patriarchy, multigenerational satanists, or space aliens that are bringing the movement to a grinding halt. It's the retractors in a court of law. With stacks of therapy notes, journals, clear memories, and evidence, retractors are taking their regressionists to court—and winning.

Dr. Chris Bardon, who is both a psychologist and an attorney, has been one of the leading figures in bringing regressionists to justice. I asked him to explain some of the common points of litigation that are being pursued in these cases. He described the following about defendants' (regressionists') liability:

1. Responsibility of a professional to provide an appropriate diagnosis.
    - Defendant negligently failed to follow appropriate guidelines for evaluating and treating patients with symptoms such as those manifested by the Plaintiff.

- Defendant failed to take a proper history from the Plaintiff.
- Defendant failed to perform appropriate examinations and diagnostic tests.
- Defendant failed to recognize Plaintiff's underlying psychiatric difficulties.

2. Responsibility of a professional to provide appropriate treatment.
   - Defendant breached standard of reasonable care expected of professionals and claimed expertise.
   - Defendant negligently failed to properly monitor Plaintiff's ongoing symptoms and the degeneration of her or his mental condition.
   - Defendant negligently failed to consult with other professionals regarding the appropriate diagnosis, evaluation, treatment, and care of Plaintiff.

3. Responsibility to use techniques appropriately and for understanding their limitations.
   - Defendant negligently misused hypnosis techniques on Plaintiff.
   - Defendant misused drugs, medications, hypnosis, and/or sodium amytal which would be expected to increase Plaintiff's responsiveness to suggestion.
   - Defendant uncritically accepted the existence of "repressed" memories of childhood sexual abuse in Plaintiff without making any effort to obtain independent verification for the truth or falsity of such "memories."
   - Defendant misapplied the concepts of "denial" and "resistance" in the treatment of Plaintiff.
   - Defendant failed to explore and/or recognize the effects of his or her own beliefs on Plaintiff.

4. Responsibility not to extend therapy unnecessarily.
   - Defendant negligently undertook and sustained a course of treatment which improperly and inappropriately extended the length of the course of Plaintiff's treatment.
   - Defendant failed to discharge Plaintiff from the hospital when it was apparent that conditions did not require inpatient treatment.

5. Responsibility to obtain informed consent from patients.

- Defendant negligently and carelessly failed to inform the Plaintiff of the risks of his or her chosen treatment techniques.
- Defendant failed to warn Plaintiff of the possibility of an adverse psychiatric condition.
- Defendant failed to advise Plaintiff that the techniques utilized had the capacity to produce false memories of events which never occurred but which nevertheless may seem real to the patient.
- Defendant failed to adequately advise Plaintiff of experimental nature of drug regime and of possible side effects of the use of prescribed psychotropic drugs in combination with others.
- Defendant failed to advise Plaintiff that the diagnosis of multiple personality disorder is controversial and that there are disputes within the mental health community as to its existence.
- Defendant failed to advise Plaintiff that a person can be taught to display behaviors of "multiple personality disorder" through the use of psychotherapy (iotrogenesis).
- Defendant dissuaded Plaintiff from seeking services from other mental health professionals or from seeking a second opinion.[18]

It's been an interesting process to watch. With warm, unconditional, positive regard for their clients, these are the professionals that argued

- Believe the victims, regardless of the lack of evidence. Questioning their claims is harmful to their psychological well being.
- Victims don't have to prove their claims in a court of law, it's their emotional reality that counts!
- The accused are assumed to be guilty and in denial about their crimes.
- The mental disorders in a client's life are proof that he or she has been abused.

But with incredible irony, once these same professionals are taken to court by their former clients (retractors), their standard becomes completely different:

- Don't believe the retractors' claims of therapy abuse, regardless of the stacks of client notes, journals, eyewitness accounts, hospital records, and other evidence they are producing. Questioning the retractor's claims must be done and is essential for the therapist's well being.
- Retractors have to prove their claims in a court of law, it's the rights of the accused therapist that count.
- Accused therapists must be presumed innocent and be afforded every legal right in defending themselves.
- The mental disorders in a retractor's life are proof that charges of therapy abuse are false.

But regardless of the regressionists' double standard, in the clear light of a court of law their exotic theories and practices are being revealed as mental-health fraud. As was the case with bringing the earlier witch-hunts to a close, the court of law has proven to be the most important arena for stopping regression hysteria and bringing its promoters to justice. A precedent setting court ruling captures the growing legal response:

"The Court finds that the testimony of the victims as to their memory of the assaults shall not be admitted at trial because the phenomenon of memory repression, and the process of therapy used in these cases to recover the memories, have not gained general acceptance in the field of psychology; and are not scientifically reliable."[19]

Toward the Future

So what happens next? Dr. Paul McHugh, director of psychiatry at Johns Hopkins University Medical School, has been very helpful in my own journey in coming to terms with the False Memory Crisis. We were recently presenters at a national conference on false memory sponsored by Johns Hopkins. In the course of the conference Dr. McHugh discussed insightful comments regarding where regressionism is headed:

The false memory epidemic is a human phenomenon of crowd behavior. Many of us have commented about the similarity of this situation to the witch trials and the lynch mobs in which anger and violence against people have been generated without evidence. It is useful to recognize that our social scientists have long since demonstrated that cultures can be swept by a craze or a false idea that takes a very standard course almost predictable in its form.

The best discussion of crazes was written in 1952 by L. S. Penrose who, in his book, *Objective Study of Crowd Behaviour*, described five different stages that crazes go through, both of an innocuous as well as a dangerous kind.

Phase I Latent Phase. Penrose defined this initial phase of the craze by stating that the idea which is the source of the problem is found in a few minds, but is not spreading. An example of this in our situation might be the idea that Multiple Personality Disorder was an expression of dissociation and child abuse that Cornelia Wilbur and a few of her associates held in the early 1970s.

Phase II Explosive Phase. During this phase the idea spreads exponentially within a community of interested people. For example, beginning in the late 1970s and early '80s the idea that repressed memories could include historical aspects of a person's life spread within much of the mental health community and took on remarkable forms, including beliefs about satanic ritual abuse and even alien abduction. The susceptibility seemed to rest upon the search for some explanation for a variety of mental disorders that are often difficult to treat. The repressed memory concept satisfied this need.

Phase III Saturation Phase. This phase is characterized by the market of "susceptible" minds in the community becoming saturated and the number of new converts to the idea slackening. It seems to me that we are in this phase with the repressed memory craze. Fewer people seem ready to immediately acquiesce to the idea. This phase, though, is difficult to distinguish from the following phase.

Phase IV Immunity Phase. This phase is characterized by resistance to the idea that develops within the community and enthusiasm weakens for it, even amongst the initially involved. Resistance develops as individuals study the idea and its implications. In our case, the study from many excellent investigators of the logic behind the concept of "repressed memories" and the shabbiness of the data that generated the ideas and supports it today provokes much of this resistance and, as has been seen by many of the initial proponents, they begin to recognize that their reputation may be damaged if they are not more careful in their advocacy of these ideas. I believe that our situation with false memories could be considered somewhere between the Phase III / Phase IV stages as outlined by Penrose.

Phase V Stagnant Phase. This phase is characterized by the idea fading away, except perhaps in the minds of a few enthusiasts. This is the place where false memories will be within the next five to ten years. The phase will be generated in part by science, but in part by legal processes in which the malpractices that generated the idea of repressed memories will be demonstrated, and eventually psychotherapeutic practices will be restored to their initial integrity. The important point is that one cannot expect everyone to see the misdirection that the repressed memory idea generated. We must accept the fact that this idea will remain in the minds of some who will become progressively more marginalized in the field of mental health by their support of these views.

I am optimistic that exactly this course is being followed but it carries the implications that we must continue our efforts to immunize the public and document as best as we can this historical moment of grief and misdirection in our field.[20]

Second Thoughts

Second thoughts are ever wiser.
EURIPIDES, *HIPPOLYTUS*, 428 B.C.

Rossell Robbins notes:

What makes witchcraft so repellent, and morally lower than fascism, is that throughout civilized Europe, in every country . . . the clergy led the persecutions and condoned them in the name of Christianity, while the lawyers and judges and professors abetted them in the name of reason. . . . The men on the side of humanity were those priests and ministers who revolted against their religion, often in the process suffering as "witch lovers," along with those skeptics labeled by their opponents as "sadducees and atheists." Shaming the cowards and addleheads, the sycophants and opportunists, these people showed the alternative way. . . . On a key issue of the sixteenth and seventeenth centuries, "Do you do or do you not approve the trials, the methods used to produce confessions, and the whole apparatus of witch hunting?" Only a few replied Nay. These men, the "witch defenders," had become the real enemy. These courageous few shook off the burden of credulity and opened the way for the age of reason and new mental horizons free from thought control. Throughout these centuries, those who should, by their birth, training, and position, have been the conscience of the world, accepted the delusion and promoted it. Such men not only appealed to the emotions of religion, but perverted the entire structure of logic and reason. Everything was sacrificed to a preconceived prejudice. The logic of the demonologists, all highly educated men, leaders in their own disciplines, is the most terrifying feature of witchcraft. Because of their turning rational thinking on its head—far more than the most foul act of a torturer or witch judge—the centuries of the witchcraft mania may be called the centuries of un civilization. . . . When the majority of educated men think in such a frame of reference, and the majority of poorly educated men follow them, humanity's chances for survival become dim. . . . Nothing about witchcraft is more ominous than the suppression and destruction of man's power to think and his right to ask questions. Those who set up the witchcraft delusion and spread it damaged Europe's culture for as long as that delusion was not rejected. Our civilization today is that much retarded.[21]

The paradigm of regressionism offered surety and comfort. It allowed its faithful believers black and white answers, satisfied "effort after meaning," promised unlimited healing and furthered the political, social and theological agendas of its promoters. But the paradigm of the recovered memory movement is falling apart. Under closer examination it simply has failed to meet the tests of science or Scripture. In the end it is being revealed as a therapeutic deception that has destroyed thousands of lives.

This much we know for sure, real abuse of children occurs. We also know that we are in the midst of an epidemic of false memories. It is not an "either/or" proposition, it is both. The only thing that compares to the horror of child abuse is to be falsely accused of these crimes. But in society's rush to judgment, the basic human right to be presumed innocent until proven guilty has often been lost. We are charged with an awesome task of finding balance, and we can accept nothing less. In finding this balance there are three principles we must keep in mind:

1. False memories are a well-documented phenomenon that occur naturally in people. Thousands have claimed forgotten incest, multigenerational satanic abuse, space alien abductions, recovered past lives or regressing into the womb. Of all these cases, it is clear that a large portion of "recovered memories" are instances of false memories. These fantasies can be the product of misinformation, therapist leading, toxic group influences, fantasy proneness, Grade Five Syndrome, personality disorders, mental illness, or faulty belief systems.

2. The theory of repression awaits evidence for its existence. Despite almost 100 years of claims by its proponents, there still is no solid evidence that has been presented. Remember our discussion in Chapter 3—the best we can determine at this time is hypnotic images draw from one of three sources: a) historical events, b) pure fantasies, or c) a bizarre mixing of historical and fantasized elements. Apart from independent, external confirmation, there is no proven way for anyone (including the accuser) to determine the true source of a hypnotic image. Even if some repressed memories are one day shown to be real, it still does not invalidate the fact that false memories are occurring for a large portion of clients and families.

3. We know that regression techniques are misleading and contribute to the creation of documented false memories. Recently I was in the mid-west for a seminar. While I was preparing for the day, I picked up the morning paper. My eyes glanced across an interesting disclaimer written over the daily horoscope—"NOTE: Horoscopes have no basis in scientific fact and should be read for entertainment, not for guidance." If only the same could be provided to those who wander into the regressionist's office. "WARNING: Regression beliefs and practices have no basis in scientific fact and should not be confused with legitimate psychotherapy. There is no demonstrated improvement for regression patients and treatment has no recognized point of termination. If you choose to proceed you should expect to lose your

mental health, grasp of reality, immediate and extended family, your career, life savings, and possibly kill yourself."

C. S. Lewis notes, "We may not be able to get certainty, but we can get probability, and half a loaf is better than no bread."[22] While there may be actual cases of repression, traumatic fantasies associated with regression therapy, readings, recovery groups and/or highly suggestible clients are less likely to be real. So I sit with my half loaf of bread, open to future evidence for repression while maintaining a healthy, caring skepticism.

I was a dutiful disciple of regression beliefs and practices—as a psychologist and a Christian I promoted this cause with the greatest sincerity. But my journey in searching for the truth took me to a radically different conclusion than my regression indoctrination had trained me in. In the final analysis, I came to understand the recovered memory movement is not about abusing white males, elusive satanists, hidden past lives, or marauding space aliens. It's about mental health fraud, unleased zeal and societal hysteria. It's about our cherished misbeliefs, deception, and a False Memory Crisis that has gripped our nation and our world.

Today, through Project Middle Ground, I continue my work to undo the wrongs that I once perpetrated on others. Despite the recent progress we've been able to make in addressing the False Memory Crisis, I'm not sure what lies around the bend. How long we will be caught in regressionism's panicked grip before we are able to free ourselves? One thing I've learned from previous hysterias is that the first ones to speak out against the injustices were seen as betraying the "cause" and labeled one of "them" and soon found themselves amongst the accused, in the coliseums, burning at the stake, in gas chambers or blacklisted. But at some point people have to stand up to hysteria's bullies and fight for a return to reason and justice. The return happens one life at a time. You and I are presented with a challenge that needs to be answered. Each of us has the power to choose. How will you respond?

A Word to Regression Believers

Experience by itself proves nothing. If a man doubts whether he is dreaming or waking, no experiment can solve his doubt, since every experiment may itself be part of the dream. Experience proves this, or that, or nothing, according to the preconceptions we bring to it.

C. S. LEWIS, *GOD IN THE DOCK*, 1942

Awake, you who sleep, arise from the dead, and Christ will give you light.

EPHESIANS 5:14

If you've experienced recovered traumatic memories and have read this far in the book, I want to thank you for hearing me out. I'm very aware things I've shared have angered and frustrated you. It isn't my wish to hurt you. But sometimes the most important gifts aren't the things we want to hear, the conclusions that agree with our own. Sometimes we need to hear the things that turn on the light, point to the doubts we've secretly held. I know that's the same thing your therapist told you when you began to recover memories. But what I'm sharing with you is not based on far-flung theories that require you to enter a special state of consciousness to understand. I'm talking common sense, reason, scriptural truths, science—things that can be openly verified by taking a trip to the library, talking with memory experts, becoming more informed, allowing yourself to ask forbidden questions.

By writing this book I am opening myself up to hostile examination and attack. Some regression believers will find fault with most everything I've said and will choose to keep seeing the world through regression lenses. This is a right they have, and they are responsible for the consequences of their choices. But I also know there are some who are still able to hear another perspective. There is a chance you are one of them. That makes the risks I've taken worthwhile. If you've read this far in the book, maybe there's a part of you that is still skeptical about your recovered memories— you're still searching for what is true. I wish I could find the words

221

that could somehow bridge the gap between you and me, a way to reach out my hand to yours and show you the way out. The best that I know to do is to speak straight and from the heart, to somehow step back into the beliefs with you for a moment and point to the exits. I was here, I stood right where you are standing, and I believed with passion and conviction. Then I discovered there was life beyond this dark valley that we've walked into. The way out doesn't lie further in, it lies behind you, back up the steep trail you've been descending.

You may feel that there's no way to turn back, you've gone too far into this, said and done too much. How could you possibly throw away the years, the money, the tears, the rage that you've invested? But stop for a moment. Catch your breath. Hear me out. What if the descent into this valley isn't necessary? What if the theories you and I were taught are wrong? There's still time to ask some hard questions. What's the rush? If what we've been taught is real, it will stand up to closer examination. If it can't, do you really want to give up your life for it?

What About the Cost?

Is this really what you had in mind when you began therapy? If I had come to you a few months before you started your therapy and told you that you were about to embark on a venture that would consume your entire life, keep you in an endless repetition of therapy and group sessions, engage you in a never-ending search for memories, make you experience constant rage, fear, hate, and isolation from lifetime family and friends, plague you with suicidal thoughts, loneliness, and blinding fear. . . . If I told you that you would step into a therapy that would go on for decades and cost you thousands of dollars, your career, and your own children. . . . Tell me, would you have gone into all this as quickly and naively as you did? Honestly, would you? Shouldn't someone have told you of the horrors that lay ahead, before you were taken in step-by-step?

When Is Therapy Finished?

Have you noticed that no one ever graduates from therapy? The further you get in, the more expansive it becomes. The readings, sessions, seminars, and groups consume more and more of your life. The old timers go on to lead groups, get degrees in counseling. But no one ever is told "You're done. You can get on with your life now." Regression therapy is like the old "No Roach Hotel" bug-catcher—"They check in but they never check out." So I'm asking, when will you know that it's time to leave therapy? Be honest now. What final memory, what final goal will have been attained that lets you know it's okay to move on? Are you really getting closer to this goal?

What Does This Feel Like from the Other Side?

Imagine what it would be like to have your grown daughter accuse you two decades from now of sexual crimes against her, crimes that you never committed but that she adamantly believes you did. The charges are never specific—you're supposed to know. Imagine how it feels to watch your child consumed in a therapeutic black hole. Everything you've ever done with her is twisted into dark events. A therapist who has never spoken with you interprets photographs as having obvious indicators that you sexually abused your daughter. The endless hours of your own therapy, which you did when she was younger, are considered "abandonment." How would you feel as you watch her repeatedly attempt suicide, move in and out of hospitals, isolate from lifelong friends and family members? In all of this she cuts off any contact from you. There is no avenue for you to defend yourself. You can only speak with her if you first confess to these crimes. But you didn't do these things! The fact that you can't recall any sexual abuse is proof that you dissociated the events. Remember, you have a dissociative disorder, which only proves that you did these crimes.

As hard as it may be for you to believe, these questions capture the reactions, the anger, horror, helplessness of your parents in the here and now. I'm talking about your real parents, the ones with real faults, strengths, flesh and blood, not the stereotypes they've been transformed into during the course of your therapy.

What About the Christian Perspective?

If you're a Christian, let me ask: How would Christ expect you to act in this situation? Not the Christ you learned in therapy—I'm talking about the Christ of the Bible. Is this really the freedom He promised you? Are the hate, rage, fear, loneliness, suicidal thoughts, and lack of functioning really fruits of the Holy Spirit?

Your therapist has told you that you have to "go through the wound in order to heal," that the devastation of your life is proof that the memories are real. I'm asking you, what if the wound is from your therapy? What if your mental breakdown isn't the product of some hidden trauma decades ago but is rather directly related to the therapy you did yesterday and the session you'll be doing tomorrow?

Are You Allowed to Think for Yourself?

What are three criticisms you have about the regression therapy you've been involved with? Stop for a moment and really answer this question. What are three things that are wrong with the regression movement? Or how about three things that you don't like about your therapist? Put the book down a second and think through your answers.

Did you have a hard time answering these questions? Maybe you didn't even put the book down. You see, you've been trained to always defend your therapist and the movement; you're not supposed to criticize the party or its doctrines. Haven't you noticed that no one in your group is allowed to speak critically of the recovered memory movement? The hypnotic images only are allowed to be real. Anything or anyone that questions is seen as the product of evil forces. The FMS Foundation is considered full of perpetrators. The mountains of research findings that contradict regressionism are always explained away. Those who doubt are part of the "old world," perpetrators, those in denial. But those who refuse to question recovered memories are the bold survivors, the ones who dare to live with the truth. Come on! Let yourself think. If no evidence is ever allowed in to challenge the things you've been taught, how will you know what parts are false teaching? Wasn't getting into therapy about learning to become independent, to break free of control, and to be able to think for yourself? What if all you've done is trade in your parents' control for control by your therapist and group members? What if you're still dancing the same dance—you've simply changed partners?

How About the Retractors?

Have you noticed that you're not allowed to have open discussions with retractors? You've been told that they've slipped back into denial, that they simply weren't strong like you and have caved in to pressure from family members. What if you told your group that you were having conversations with a retractor? Would they approve? Here's an idea—dare to talk with one and hear why she or he got out. You'll find articulate women and men who have been through therapeutic hell and come out the other side. With clarity, anger, and relief they'll share their experiences. They're a far cry from the stereotypes you've been taught. Remember, one of the things you object to is people who haven't taken the time to talk to you, to understand your situation before they've decided your memories are false. Don't retractors deserve the same courtesy?

Can You Question Any of the Memories?

How can someone tell if her "memories" are actually fantasies? If someone came to you with vivid, detailed memories of being tortured in former lives, what would you say to her? Would you be allowed to question her reality? She explains that she's felt much better since she found out she was murdered as a slave in Egypt. What if it was about space aliens? How would you respond? If you had doubts about the truth of her memories and somehow found the freedom to speak freely, what would you say to help her? What if you simply questioned the reality of some of your own memories? Honestly now, do you really think your therapist and group members would allow you to do that? Would they accept you if you decided that a portion of your memories was false? You've spent so much time learning how to affirm abusive memories as true—how to define every symptom a person has, how to read every conceivable reaction of the accused. Honestly, do you believe all the recovered memories are real? Are your sexual abuse or other violent memories real, or are they just believable? How would you know which is which? If you're not allowed to question any of your memories, how will you ever know which is which?

The bottom line is that many former clients are discovering they've been mind-raped by regression's teachings and practices. They're not crazy, in denial, or running from the truth. They've simply figured out that they were able to imagine things that were suggested or read to them. Their problems began when authorities in their lives insisted that their fantasies could only be real. Their escape finally came when they allowed themselves to question their indoctrination, to step back and see their fantasies from another perspective. They dared to think for themselves, to ask the questions that had been denied them by therapists and group members. Maybe, just maybe, this is your story as well.

The good news is that your recovered memories don't have to be real. You can choose which way your life is headed. But in choosing, take the time to verify that the events and teachings you are basing your decisions upon stand up to rigorous examination.

In the course of your treatment you've been told that you have a number of rights. "You don't have to prove your memories to anyone but yourself." "Your emotional reality is all that counts." "You don't have to justify cutting people out of your life, you're an adult who can choose." Let me share with you some additional rights, ones that you may not have been told about:

1) You have a right to competent therapy that is based on science and reflects the state-of-the-art understanding about the human condition. You have a right to be free of your therapist's hang-ups and agendas, false beliefs, and misinformation.

2) You have the right to know that regression teachings, symptoms lists, and trauma models of memory are theories which haven't been scientifically validated. You have the right to be fully informed (in writing) about the experimental nature of regression techniques, their scientifically demonstrated delusional affects, and the cautions that professional organizations have issued against recovered memory therapy.

3) You also have the right to know that clients who are subjected to these teachings and techniques consistently experience severe psychological decompensation. There are no scientific studies which demonstrate that clients are better once they've gone through regressionism. In fact, the evidence shows that clients' lives are much worse.

4) If you are working with a Christian therapist you have a right to a truthful presentation of Scripture. It is not okay for your therapist to misrepresent or distort various Scriptures in an attempt to manipulate you or imply that repressionism is a biblical notion. You have a right to know that "Holy Spirit techniques" for memory recovery are actually standard hypnotic inductions which have simply been renamed.

5) You have the right to know that without solid, external evidence, there is no way for you or your therapist to determine whether your hypnotic images are historical, pure fantasy, or some combination of the two. It is unprofessional and irresponsible for your therapist to assert that your recovered memories can only be real.

6) You have the right to feel positive about your therapist and group members but determine that some portion of what you are being taught is false, misleading, or manipulative. To do so does not mean you are rejecting them or blaspheming God. It's okay to realize that they've been working under some common misconceptions in a sincere effort to help you. It isn't okay for your therapist or group members to threaten you, shame you, tell you you're blaspheming against the Holy Spirit, say you're in denial, or insinuate that you're perpetrating against your own children or other group members. You don't have to accept their all-or-nothing expectations.

7) You have a right to read false memory research and books, and have open discussions with those who are addressing the False Memory Crisis. You have a right to know that false memories are a proven, scientific fact that may have relevance to your situation. You also have the right to talk with retractors and discover why they got out of regressionism. They have their own stories, which warrant a fair hearing. They deserve the same respect and opportunity that you expect for yourself and other regression believers.

8) You have the right to take a vacation from therapy. Remember, this was therapy that *you* initiated, and you are the consumer who is investing time, energy, and finances. At any time you have the right to decide to take a break from your therapist and groups to simply be quiet, check out other perspectives, save your money, or redirect your energies.

9) You have the right to open up lines of communication with family members who do not believe your memories. It is okay to speak with the accused—they do not have to confess before you are allowed to be in contact with them again. You may think that your parents and siblings will have nothing to

do with you after so much has transpired. You might be right, but then again you might be wrong. You won't know until you try opening the door. It may be closed on the other side. At least you'll know either way.

Plenty of families are imperfect. Realizing that some of your recovered memories are false doesn't mean that you must deny the reality of everything that was hurtful. There are lots of retractors who will tell you they grew up in harmful relationships, experiencing sexual abuse, controlling fathers, distant mothers, and so on. Retractors simply came back to the reality that they always knew—both the good and the bad—and are working to heal from that point forward.

You don't have to recant; you don't have to make some kind of public confession. Think of a way to open up some limited, safe contact. Allow for an exchange of letters or limited phone calls; meet with them in a neutral place with a friend there to support you. Agree to disagree—if they don't insist that you're wrong, then you can do the same for them. Maybe you can't have 100 percent of a relationship, but how about 30 percent? It's a start, and maybe that's far enough for a lifetime. One step, one foot in front of the other. The days are turning into weeks, into months, into years. Holidays, family gatherings, weddings, funerals are coming and going. The moments that make for a lifetime of relationships are falling away, one petal at a time, and they don't come back. When your parents are dead, when nieces and nephews are graduated and married, when lives have moved on, only then will the fruit of what you've planted and nurtured day after day be fully realized.

Remember Mary's story, the one that started this book? I asked her a simple question: What would you tell people who are still caught up in regression beliefs? She shared with me the following:

Imagine going to the doctor's office with a broken arm. You're in a great deal of pain, expecting to find relief and healing. Your doctor asks you to fill out a medical history, and that's typical, so you agree. He finally returns to your room with your medical history in hand, but instead of tending to your arm, he sits down and begins to expound on the fact that you had chicken pox at age seven and the flu several times when you were eleven. Then he takes great interest in your dad's high blood pressure and the fact that your mom is overweight. He shares with you that your past is crucial in understanding how you came to break your arm in the present and must be better understood before he can heal it. He understands that your arm is hurting and tells you it'll get worse before it gets better, but this is the way to complete healing. He rises, hands you several books to read, a stack of questionnaires, schedules appointments for the next several weeks, and before he leaves says, "Be careful with that arm, it's very vulnerable."

Sound familiar? Do you know what happens to broken arms if they are not set and allowed to heal properly? And what about that "broken arm," the one you went to therapy for to begin with? How is it? Is it healed? And if by chance it is, did you have to break something else to find that healing? Do you have an infection? Are you whole yet? Honestly, are you really whole yet? How much longer?

The question to me doesn't have to do with "memories," "multiple personalities," a "controlling father," or a "manipulative mother." If you want to see the world through those glasses, that's your decision and your right. My question is, "Are you better now than when you started therapy?" Is that original problem that you had the insight, the courage, and the strength to seek help for better?

We know that when we go to the doctor there will be a price, but we go prepared to pay it. For your therapy there was a cost. Have you gotten what you paid for? When you started, did you ever dream that it would cost you your family, your friends, your joy, your past? Have you sacrificed your life at their altar in hopes they'd give you a new one? Would they still accept you if you questioned their reality? Honestly now, would they let you think differently from what they've taught you?

Wholeness. Liberty. New life. Hope. There are people who go through life never believing in any of those things, but not you. The very fact that you sought help to begin with shows you're a believer in something bigger than yourself, you're teachable, you're strong, and you're a fighter.

The thing you seek can be found. It's okay to look, and to keep looking, but there is a way to find what you're searching for without paying the price they've demanded of you. There is a God in heaven who loves you and who sent you His Son to give you the life you seek. He won't require you to hurt others to have it—only powerless people ask you to do that sort of thing. No insurance forms, no co-payments, and you don't find it through the past. If you follow *His* teaching, not the therapists', not the books, not the seminars or theories, but *His teaching*, then you will know the truth, and His truth will set you free!

Are you tired—or is *weary* a better word? Well, imagine being in that same doctor's office with the door shut. You feel trapped, you're banging on the walls, afraid you can't get out, and your arm really hurts. Check the knob—it's not locked. You can get out of there. A second opinion won't hurt anything. Remember, you were the one who had the strength, the courage, and the hope to open this door to begin with. The Great Physician calls. He's standing, knocking.

Turn the knob.

It's not locked.

At least get that arm looked at.

Notes

Chapter 1.   Second Thoughts

1. C. S. Lewis, *Poems*, edited by Walter Hooper (New York: Harcourt Brace Jovanovich, 1964).
2. Rosanne Barr, "A Star Cries Incest," *People*, 7 October 1991, 84-88.
3. Marilyn Van Derbur, "The Darkest Secret," *People*, 10 June 1991, 89-94.
4. Advertisement in *Changes* Magazine, October 1992.
5. Ibid.
6. Ibid.
7. Chauncey Hollingsworth, "Pyschiatrist Looks to Patients' Past Lives for Cures," *the Arizona Daily Star*, 30 June 1995, Section D, page 2.
8. Ibid.
9. Ibid.
10. ABC's *20/20* show, "Regression Therapy: Have You Been There Before?" by Hugh Downs, 10/29/93.
11. Marjorie Rosen, J. D. Podolsky, and S. Avery Brown, "Out of This World," *People*, 23 May 1994.
12. Ibid.
13. Ibid.
14. Ibid.
15. Ibid.
16. Ibid.
17. Ibid.
18. Calculation given by Carl Sagan, "What's Really Going On?" *Parade*, March 7, 1993, 4-7. This was in response to findings by Bud Hopkins, David Michael Jacobs, and Ron Westrum, "Unusual Personal Experiences," *The Roper Organization*, (1992), 1-59.
19. "Divided Memories, Part 1—The Hunt for Memory," *Frontline*, Ofra Bikel show #1312, WGBH Educational Foundation, 4 April 1995.
20. Michael Yapko, *Suggestions of Abuse* (New York: Simon & Schuster, 1994), 57.
21. *The Oprah Winfrey Show*, "Womb Regression," 7/13/94.
22. D. A. Poole, D. S. Memon and R. Bull, "Psychotherapy and the Recovery of Memories of Childhood Sexual Abuse: U.S. and British Practioner's Opinions, Practices, and Experiences," *Journal of Consulting and Clinical Psychology*, 63 (1995), 426-437.
23. *The Oprah Winfrey Show*, 10/2/89. Quoted by Joe Salkowski, "A Different Diagnosis," the *Arizona Daily Star*, 5 December 1994, Section A, 9.
24. Michael Yapko, *Suggestions of Abuse* (New York: Simon & Schuster, 1994), 54.

25. American Medical Association, "Memories of Childhood Abuse," *Report of the Council on Scientific Affairs*, CSA Report 5-A-94, 1994, 4.

Chapter 2. The World of Regressionism

1. "Divided Memories, Part 1."

2. Elizabeth Loftus and Katherine Ketcham, *The Myth of Repressed Memory* (New York: St. Martin's Press, 1994), 49. Reprinted with permission by St. Martin's Incorporated.

3. Sigmund Freud, Repression. *"The Standard Edition of the Complete Psychological Works of Sigmund Freud*, ed. Jo Strachey, vol. 14 (London: Hogarth, 1957), 16.

4. Peter Gay, *The Freud Reader* (New York: W.W. Norton 1989), 103.

5. Richie Herink, ed., preface. *The Psychotherapy Handbook* (New York: New American Library, 1980),

6. Brochure mailed to the author.

7. See Gary Almy and Carol Tharp Almy, *Addicted to Recovery* (Harvest House, 1994) and Ed Bulkley *Why Christians Can't Trust Psychology* (Harvest House, 1993) for an expansion on political and social agendas of modern psychology.

8. The most recent title for Multiple Personality Disorder in the *DSM-IV* is "Dissociative Personality Disorder" or "DID." In this book I've chosen to continue with the use of "MPD" in order to lessen confusion for the reader.

9. Morey Bernstein, *The Search for Bridey Murphy* (Garden City, N.Y.: Doubleday, 1956).

10. E. Bass and L. Davis, *The Courage to Heal: A Guide for Women Survivors of Child Sexual Abuse* (New York: Harper & Row, 1988), 21.

11. Ibid., 22.

12. Ibid., 81.

13. Ibid., 347.

14. Gay, *The Freud Reader*, 103.

15. Joe Salkowski, "A Different Diagnosis," *The Arizona Daily Star*, 5 December 1994, sec. A.

16. Ibid.

17. Ibid.

18. Yapko, *Suggestions of Abuse* 54.

19. Ibid., 54.

20. Gay, *The Freud Reader*, 112.

21. Gay, *The Freud Reader*, 113.

Chapter 3. Repression Takes The Stand

1. Joe Salkowski, "Deadly Memories," *The Arizona Daily Star*, 6 December 1994, Sec. A.
2. Ibid.
3. Ibid.
4. Ibid.
5. Ibid.
6. C. S. Lewis, *God in the Dock: Essays on Theology and Ethics*. ed. Walter Hooper (Grand Raids: Eerdmans, 1970), 11–112.
7. Hollingsworth, "Pyschiatrist Looks to Patients' Past Lives For Cures."
8. Ibid.
9. Judith Lewis Herman and Emily Schatzow, "Recovery and Verification of Memories of Childhood Sexual Trauma," *Psychoanalytic Psychology*, 4, 1 (1987): 1–14.
10. Joe Salkowski, "Out of the Dark," *The Arizona Daily Star*, 4 December 1994, sec. A.
11. Ibid.
12. John Briere and Jon Conte, "Amnesia in Adults Molested as Children," (paper presented at the annual meeting of the American Psychological Association, New Orleans, August 1989). Later published as, "Self-Reported Amnesia for Abuse in Adults Molested as Children," *Journal of Traumatic Stress*, 6. 1 (1993), 21–31.
13. Linda Williams, "Adult Memories of Childhood Abuse: Preliminary Findings From a Longitudinal Study," *APSAC Advisor* (summer), 19–21.
14. Donna Della Femina, Catherine A. Yeager, and Dorothy Otnow Lewis, "Child Abuse: Adolescent Records vs. Adult Recall," *Child Abuse and Neglect*, 14 (1990): 227–231.
15. New Hampshire v. Joel Hungerford, 94-045 thru 94-S-047; State of New Hampshire v. John Morahan, 93-S-1734 thru 93-S-1936, (1994).
16. Associated Press, "5-year Old's Secret Kept for 29 Years Convicts Father of Murdering Mother," *The Arizona Daily Star*, 20 April 1995, sec. A.
17. Associated Press, "Woman's Nightmare Nears End," *The Arizona Daily Star*, 15 July 1995, sec. B.
18. M. L. Howe, M. L. Courage and C. Peterson, "Intrusions in Preschoolers' Recall of Traumatic Childhood Events," *Psychonomic Bulletin & Review*, 2. 1 (1995), 130–134. Also see their earlier paper, "Children's Memories of Traumatic Events," (presented at the annual meeting of the *Psychonomic Society*, St. Louis, Mi, November, 1994).
19. C. P. Malmquist, "Children Who Witness Parental Murder: Postraumatic Aspects," *Journal of the American Academy of Child Psychiatry*, 25, 3 (1986): 320–325.
20. C. Safran, "Dangerous Obsession: The Truth about Repressed Memories," *McCall's*, June 1993, 98–155.

21. Dr. Paul McHugh, personal communication with the author.
22. William A. Wagenaar and Joe Groeneweg, "The Memory of Concentration Camp Survivors," *Applied Cognitive Psychology*, 4 (1990): 77.
23. *State of New Hampshire v. Joel Hungerford, State of New Hampshire v. John Morahan*
24. David Holmes, "The Evidence for Repression: An Examination of Sixty Years of Research," *Repression and Dissociation*, Ed. Jerome L. Singer (Chicago: The Univ. of Chicago Press, 1990), 96–98.
25. "Scientific Status of Refreshing Recollection by the Use of Hypnosis," *Journal of the American Medical Association*, 253, (5 April 1985): 1922. *Resolution 504-Misuse of Hypnosis and Other Techniques of "Memory Enhancement/Creation"* (June 1993). American Medical Association, "Memories of Childhood Abuse," *Report of the Council on Scientific Affairs*, CSA Report 5-A-94 (16 June 1994).
26. C. S. Lewis, *An Experiment in Criticism* (Cambridge: Cambridge Univ. Press, 1961), 56.
27. Calculation by Carl Sagan, "What's Really Going On?,"
28. Lewis, *God in the Dock* 111–112.

Chapter 4. Stumbling Down Memory Lane

1. For an excellent discussion on this subject see J. O'Sullivan and M. Howe, "Metamemory and Memory Construction," *Consciousness and Cognition*, 4 (1995): 104–110.
2. U. Neisser and N. Harsch, "Phantom Flashbulbs: False Recollections of Hearing the News about Challenger," *Affect and Accuracy in Recall: Studies of "Flashbulb Memories*, ed. E. Winograd and U. Neisser (Cambridge, U.K.: Cambridge Univ. Press, 1992).
3. E. F. Loftus and K. Ketcham, *Witness for the Defense* (New York: St. Martin's Press, 1991), 20. Reprinted with permission by St. Martin's Incorporated.
4. This is a composite story.
5. Salkowski, "A Different Diagnosis."
6. Ibid.
7. Ibid.
8. Ibid.
9. Client's story (altered).
10. Dr. Paul Ingmundson, personal communication to the author.
11. Yapko, *Suggestions of Abuse*, 57.
12. Pamela Freyd, "The False Memory Syndrome Foundation: Response to a Mental Health Crisis," (to appear in: Halperin, D.A. (Ed.), *False Memory Syndrome: Therapeutic and Forensic Perspectives*. American Psychiatric Press, forthcoming).
13. See the following studies by D. B. Pillemer and S. H. White, "Childhood Events Recalled by Children and Adults," *Advances in*

Child Development and Behavior, Vol. 21. (New York: Academic Press, 1989). Also, E. Winograd, E. and W.A. Killinger, "Relating Age at Encoding in Early Childhood to Adult Recall: Development of Flashbulb Memories," *Journal of Experimental Psychology: General* (1983): 112, 413–422. Finally, Sheingold and Tenney, "Memory for a Salient Childhood Event," *Memory Observed*, ed. U. Neisser (San Francisco: Freeman, 1982), 201-212.

14. Salkowski, "A Different Diagnosis."

15. Nicholas P. Spanos, Evelyn Menary, Natalie J. Gabora, Susan C. DuBreuil, and Bridget Dewhirst, "Secondary Identity Enactments During Hypnotic Past-Life Regression: A Sociocognitive Perspective," *Journal of Personality and Social Psychology* 61, 2 (1991): 308.

16. Loftus and Ketcham, *The Myth of Repressed Memory* 73–101.

17. Richard Ofshe and Ethan Watters, *Making Monsters* (New York: Charles Scribner's Sons, 1994), 155–176.

18. Peter J. Reveen, Fantasizing under Hypnosis: Some Experimental Evidence, *The Skeptical Inquirer*, Vol. 12, (Winter 1987), 181–182.

19. Nicholas P. Spanos, Patricia A. Cross, Kirby Dickson, and Susan C. DuBreuil, "Close Encounters: An Examination of UFO Experiences," *Journal of Abnormal Psychology*, 102, 4 (1993): 624–632.

Chapter 5. Satanic Panic

1. This retractor's story has been changed (her name and certain identifying features) to protect her identity.

2. Special acknowledgments to Zachary Bravos, "Child Abuse and Witchcraft?", *Issues in Child Abuse Accusations*, 3, 3 (1991): 144–153.

3. Rossell Robbins, *The Encyclopedia of Witchcraft and Demonology* (Crown Publishers, Inc., 1959), 13–14.

4. Randy Emon, personal communication to the author.

5. Kenneth V. Lanning, *Investigator's Guide to Allegations of "Ritual" Child Abuse*, Behavioral Science Unit, National Center for the Analysis of Violent Crime, Federal Bureau of Investigation, FBI Academy, Quantico, Virginia 22135, January 1992. Also see Kenneth V. Lanning, "Ritual Abuse: A Law Enforcement View or Perspective," *Child Abuse & Neglect*, 15, 171-173.

6. Joel Best, Missing Children, Misleading Statistics, *The Public Interest*, p. 85. Also see James Richardson, Joel Best, and David Bromley, *The Satanism Scare* (New York Aldine de Gruyter, 1991) and Bob and Gretchen Passantino, "The Facts About Satanic Ritual Abuse," *Christian Research Journal*, Winter (1992), 33.

7. Bob and Gretchen Passantino, "The Facts About Satanic Ritual Abuse," *Christian Research Journal*, Winter (1992), 33.

8. Statistic attributed to Dr. Al Carlisle of the Utah State Prison System by Jerry Johnston, *The Edge of Evil* (Dallas: Word Books, 1989).

9. Bob and Gretchen Passantino, "The Facts About Satanic Ritual Abuse," *Christian Research Journal*, Winter (1992), 33.
10. U.S. Department of Justice, *National Incidence Studies On Missing, Abducted, Runaway, and Thrownaway Children in America*, Washington, D.C. (1990).
11. Susan Lockamay Norman, "Ritual Abuse: Myth or Mystery?," *Charisma Magazine*, November 1992, 76-78.
12. Goodman, Gail S., et al., (1994). "Characteristics and Sources of Allegations of Ritualistic Child Abuse", Grant No. 90CA1405. Dr. Gail S. Goodman / Department of Psychology / University of California, Davis / Young Hall / Davis, CA 95616. This is the researchers being quoted by Daniel Goleman, "Proof Lacking for Ritual Abuse by Satanists", *the New York Times*, 31 October 1994, Section A, 13.
13. Daniel Goleman, "Proof Lacking for Ritual Abuse by Satanists", *the New York Times*, 31 October 1994, Section A, 13.
14. Ibid.
15. Ibid.
16. Ibid.
17. Ibid.
18. Ibid.
19. Kapferer, Jean-Noel, *Rumors* (New Brunswick: Transaction Publishers, 1990), 21.
20. Gregory Lewis, "Snapple Plans Ad Blitz to Rebut 'Outrageous' Klantie Rumors," *The Arizona Republic*. 2 September 1993, Section A.
21. Rossell Robbins, *The Encyclopedia of Witchcraft and Demonology* (Crown Publishers, Inc., 1959), 236.

Chapter 6. What's Your Sign?

1. Annual Texas State FMS Foundation Conference in Dallas August 26, 1994. This story is printed with Amy Smith's permission.
2. E. Sue Blume, *Secret Survivors* (New York: Ballantine Books, 1991), preface.
3. Ibid.
4. Ibid.
5. Ibid.
6. Ibid.
7. Eric L. Nelson and Paul Simpson, "First Glimpse: An Initial Examination of Subjects Who Have Rejected Their Recovered Visualization as False Memories," *Issues in Child Abuse Accusations*, Vol. 6, 3 (1994), 125.
8. Ibid., 125.
9. Ibid., 127.
10. Bud Hopkins, David Michael Jacobs, and Ron Westrum, "Unusual Personal Experiences," *The Roper Organization* (1992), 1-59.

11. Ibid.
12. Ibid., 8.
13. Calculation given by Carl Sagan, "What's Really Going On?," *Parade*, March 7, 1993, 4-7. This was in response to findings by Bud Hopkins, David Michael Jacobs, and Ron Westrum, "Unusual Personal Experiences," The Roper Organization, (1992), 1-59.
14. Brian L. Weiss, *Through Time into Healing* (New York: Simon & Schuster, 1992), 23.
15. Daniel Ryder, *Breaking the Circle of Satanic Ritual Abuse* (Minneapolis: CompCare Publishers, 1992), 67-75.
16. Ibid.
17. R. W. London, "Therapeutic Treatment of Patients with Repressed Memories," *The Independent Practitioner*, 15, No. 2 (1995, Spring), 64–67.
18. American Psychological Association (November 11, 1994), "APA Panel Addresses Controversy Over Adult Memories of Childhood Sexual Abuse" (news release).
19. Peter Gay, *The Freud Reader* (New York, W. W. Norton & Company, 1989), 100.
20. Rossell Robbins, *The Encyclopedia of Witchcraft and Demonology* (Crown Publishers, Inc., 1959), 182.
21. Ibid., 17-18.
22. Ibid., 52. Reprinted by permission of Crown Publishers, Inc.
23. American Psychiatric Association, "*Statement on Memories of Sexual Abuse*" (news release, 1993), American Psychiatric Association, 1400 K Street, NW, Washington, D. C. 20005.
24. Peter Gay, *The Freud Reader*, 103.
25. Rossell Robbins, *The Encyclopedia of Witchcraft and Demonology*, 106.
26. Personal communication from Bob and Gretchen Passantino to the author.

Chapter 7. Coming Clean

1. New Hampshire, State of. Hillsborough County Superior Court, *State of New Hampshire v. Joel Hungerford*, 94-045 thru 94-S-047, *State of New Hampshire v. John Morahan*, 93-S-1734 thru 93-S-1936 (1994), 9.
2. John F. Kihlstrom, "The Recovery of Memory in the Laboratory and Clinic", unpublished pape April 19, 1993. Later used in a chapter of *Truth and Memory*, edited by S. J. Lynn and N. P. Spanos forthcoming from Guilford Press (New York).
3. FMS Foundation, "Family Survey," presented at the 1st National Conference on FMS, *Memory & Reality: Emerging Crisis*, April 16-18, 1993.
4. This statistic is part of the findings from a recently completed study from the Washington State Department of Labor and Industries. The preliminary results are given in the *FMS Foundation Newsletter*, May 1, 1996. Personal correspondance was also shared with the author.

5. Pamela Freyd, "The False Memory Syndrome Foundation: Response to a Mental Health Crisis" (to appear in: Halperin, D.A. (Ed.), *False Memory Syndrome: Therapeutic and Forensic Perspectives*. American Psychiatric Press), 11.
6. Findings from a recently completed study from the Washington State Department of Labor and Industries. The preliminary results are given in the *FMS Foundation Newsletter*, May 1, 1996. Personal correspondence was also shared with the author.
7. FMS Foundation, "Family Survey."
8. Ibid. Also updated information from Pamela Freyd, "The False Memory Syndrome Foundation: Response to a Mental Health Crisis" (to appear in: Halperin, D.A. (Ed.), *False Memory Syndrome: Therapeutic and Forensic Perspectives*. American Psychiatric Press), 11.
9. FMS Foundation, "Family Survey."
10. Pamela Freyd, "The False Memory Syndrome Foundation: Response to a Mental Health Crisis," 12.
11. Ibid., 11.
12. FMS Foundation, "Family Survey."
13. Ibid.
14. Ibid.
15. Thomas Kuhn, *The Structure of Scientific Revolutions* (Madison: University of Wisconsin Press, 1958), 24.
16. Ibid., 94.

Chapter 8. Follow the Leader

1. Summary of several media accounts.
2. Nicholas P. Spanos, Evelyn Menary, Natalie J. Gabora, Susan C. DuBreuil, and Bridget Dewhirst, "Secondary Identity Enactments During Hypnotic Past-Life Regression: A Sociocognitive Perspective," *Journal of Personality and Social Psychology*, Vol. 61, 2 (1991), 308.
3. Nicholas P. Spanos, Patricia A. Cross, Kirby Dickson, and Susan C. DuBreuil, "Close Encounters: An Examination of UFO Experiences," *Journal of Abnormal Psychology*, Vol. 102, 4 (1993), 624.
4. Daniel Goleman, "Therapists Often Victims, Study Finds," the *Arizona Daily Star*, 23 September 1992, Section A, 5.
5. Helene Jackson and Ronald Nuttall, "Clinician Responses to Sexual Abuse Allegations," *Child Abuse & Neglect*, Vol. 17 (1993), 127-143.
6. Ibid.
7. Shirley Feldman-Summers and Kenneth S. Pope, "The Experience of 'Forgetting' Childhood Abuse: A National Survey of Psychologists," *Journal of Counseling and Clinical Psychology*, Vol. 62, 3 (1994), 636.
8. American Medical Association, Report of the Council on Scientific Affairs, *Memories of Childhood Abuse*, CSA Report 5-A-94 (June 16, 1994), 3.

9. Eric L. Nelson and Paul Simpson, "First Glimpse: An Initial Examination of Subjects Who Have Rejected Their Recovered Visualization as False Memories," *Issues in Child Abuse Accusations*, Vol. 6, 3 (1994), 127.
10. Ibid.
11. Ibid.
12. Ibid.
13. Michael D. Yapko, "Suggestibility and Repressed Memories of Abuse: A Survey of Psychotherapists' Beliefs," *American Journal of Clinical Hypnosis*, 36:3 (1994), 57.
14. Joe Salkowski, "A Different Diagnosis," the *Arizona Daily Star*, 5 December 1994, Section A, 8.
15. American Medical Association, Council on Scientific Affairs, "Scientific Status of Refreshing Recollection by the Use of Hypnosis," *Journal of the American Medical Association*, Vol. 253 (April 5, 1985), 1921.
16. Peter J. Reveen, "Fantasizing Under Hypnosis: Some Experimental Evidence," *The Skeptical Inquirer*, Vol. 12, Winter (1987), 182-183.
17. Nicholas P. Spanos, Patricia A. Cross, Kirby Dickson, and Susan C. DuBreuil, "Close Encounters: An Examination of UFO Experiences," 624.
18. Michael D. Yapko, "Suggestibility and Repressed Memories of Abuse: A Survey of Psychotherapists' Beliefs," 57.
19. American Medical Association, Council on Scientific Affairs, "Scientific Status of Refreshing Recollection by the Use of Hypnosis," 1922. See the following studies and reports concerning the parameters of hypnosis: American Medical Association, Council on Scientific Affairs, "Scientific Status of Refreshing Recollection by the Use of Hypnosis," *Journal of the American Medical Association*, Vol. 253 (April 5, 1985). American Medical Association, House of Delegates, Resolution 504—Misuse of Hypnosis and Other Techniques of "Memory Enhancement/Creation" (June 1993). American Medical Association, Report of the Council on Scientific Affairs, "Memories of Childhood abuse," *CSA Report 5-A-94* (June 16, 1994). A. Barnier K. McConkey, "Reports of Real and False Memories The Relevance of Hypnosis, Hypnotizability, and Context of Memory Test," *Journal of Abnormal Psychology*, 101(3) (1992), 521-526. E. Cardena D. Spiegel, "Suggestibility, Absorption, and Dissociation." In J. F. Schmaker (Ed.), *Human Suggestibility* (New York: Routledge, 1991), 93-107. G. K. Ganaway (1991, August 19). "Alternative Hypothesis Regarding Satanic Ritual Abuse Memories." Presented at the 99th annual convention of American Psychological Association, San Francisco, CA (August 19, 1991). John F. Kihlstrom, "The Recovery of Memory in the Laboratory and Clinic", unpublished paper April 19, 1993. Later used in a chapter of *Truth and Memory*, edited by S. J. Lynn and N. P. Spanos, forthcoming from Guilford Press (New York). M. T. Orne,

D. A. Soskis, D. F. Dinges, E. C. Orne, M. H. Tonry, "Hypnotically Refreshed Testimony: Enhanced Memory or Tampering with Evidence?" (Washington, D.C.: U.S. Dept. of Justice, National Institute of Justice, 1985). F. W. Putnam, "Dissociative Phenomena." In A. Tassman S. M. Goldfinger (Ed.). *Review of Psychiatry* (Washington, D.C.: American Psychiatric Press, 1991), 145-160. P. Sheehan, P, et al., "Pseudomemory Effects and Their Relationship to Level of Susceptibility to Hypnosis and State Instruction," *Journal of Personality and Social Psychology*, Vol. 80 (1) (January 1991), 130-137. N. P. Spanos, C. A. Quigley, M. I. Gwynn, R. L. Glatt, A. H. Perlini, "Hypnotic Interrogation, Pretrial Preparation, and Witness Testimony During Direct and Cross Examination," *Law and Human Behavior*, 15 (1991), 639-653. H. Spiegel, "The Grade 5 Syndrome: The Highly Hypnotizable Person," *The International Journal of Clinical and Experimental Hypnosis*, Vol. XXII, No. 4 (1974), 303-319.

20. New Hampshire, State of. Hillsborough County Superior Court, *State of New Hampshire v. Joel Hungerford*, 94-045 thru 94-S-047, *State of New Hampshire v. John Morahan*, 93-S-1734 thru 93-S-1936 (1994), 10–11.

Chapter 9. Join the Club

1. Eric L. Nelson and Paul Simpson, "First Glimpse: An Initial Examination of Subjects Who Have Rejected Their Recovered Visualization as False Memories," *Issues in Child Abuse Accusations*, Vol. 6, 3 (1994), 126.
2. Ibid., 127.
3. Ibid.
4. Ibid.
5. M. Sherif, "A Study of Some Social Factors in Perception," *Archives of Psychology*, 187 (1935), 60.
6. S. Asch, "Studies of Independence and Conformity," *Psychological Monographs*, 70 (1956), 9.
7. Bob Fellows, *Easily Fooled* (Minneapolis: Mind Matters, P.O. Box 16557, Minneapolis, MN 55416, 1989), 13.
8. Jack Leggett, interviewed for *Frontline*'s, "Search for Satan," WGBH Educational Foundation, Show #1402, Oct. 24, 1995.
9. Steven Hassan, *Combatting Cult Mind Control* (Rochester, Vermont: Park Street Press, 1988).
10. Ibid., 69.
11. Eric L. Nelson and Paul Simpson, "First Glimpse: An Initial Examination of Subjects Who Have Rejected Their Recovered Visualization as False Memories," 126.
12. Ibid.
13. E. Bass and L. Davis, *The Courage to Heal: A Guide for Women Survivors of Child Sexual Abuse* (New York: Harper & Row, 1988), 188-190.

14. Eric L. Nelson and Paul Simpson, "First Glimpse: An Initial Examination of Subjects Who Have Rejected Their Recovered Visualization as False Memories," 127.

15. Ibid., 125.

16. Ibid.

17. Ibid.

18. Ibid.

19. Ibid., 128.

20. Ibid., 126.

21. Steven Hassan, *Combatting Cult Mind Control*, 82.

Chapter 10. Monsters from Within

1. Personal communication from Diana Anderson to the author. See also, Joe Salkowski, "A Different Diagnosis," the *Arizona Daily Star*, 4 December 1994, Section A, 1.

2. Ibid.

3. Ibid.

4. Ibid.

5. Ibid.

6. Ibid.

7. Ibid.

8. Sheryl C. Wilson and Theodore X. Barber, "The Fantasy-Prone Personality: Implications for Understanding Imagery, Hypnosis, and Parapsychological Phenomena," chapter in *Imagery*, edited by Anees A. Sheikh (New York: John Wiley & Sons, 1983), 373-374. See also, Judith W. Rhue and Steven Jay Lynn, "Fantasy Proneness and Psychopathology," *Journal of Personality and Social Psychology*, Vol. 53, 2 (1987).

9. Sheryl C. Wilson and Theodore X. Barber, "The Fantasy-Prone Personality: Implications for Understanding Imagery, Hypnosis, and Parapsychological Phenomena," 373-374.

10. Ibid., 365-367.

11. Ibid., 377.

12. Robert E. Bartholomew, Keith Basterfield, and George S. Howard, "UFO Abductees and Contactees: Psychopathology or Fantasy Proneness?," *Professional Psychology: Research and Practice*, Vol. 22, 3 (1991), 215-222.

13. Herbert Spiegel, "The Grade 5 Syndrome: The Highly Hypnotizable Person," *The International Journal of Clinical and Experimental Hypnosis*, Vol. XXII, 4 (1974), 303-319.

14. Jon Trott, "The Grade Five Syndrome," *Cornerstone*, Vol. 20, 96 (December 1991), 16.

15. Sherrill Mulhern, "Satanism and Psychotherapy," in *The Satanism Scare*. Ed. James T. Richardson, Joel Best, and David G. Bromley (New York: Aldine de Gruyter, 1991), 148.

16. George K. Ganaway, "Historical Versus Narrative Truth: Clarifying the Role of Exogenous Trauma in the Etiology of MPD and Its Variants," *Dissociation*, 2, 4 (December 1989), 208. Quoted in Jon Trott, "The Grade Five Syndrome," *Cornerstone*, Vol. 20, 96 (December 1991), 16.
17. Jon Trott, "The Grade Five Syndrome," 16.
18. Ibid.
19. *Diagnostic and Statistical Manual of Mental Disorders, Fourth Edition*, American Psychiatric Assoication, 1994, 479-481.
20. Ibid., 485-486.
21. Jon Trott, "The Grade Five Syndrome," 18.
22. Paul Brand and Philip Yancey, *Pain: The Gift Nobody Wants* (New York: Harper Collins, 1993), 211-212.
23. Eric L. Nelson and Paul Simpson, "First Glimpse: An Initial Examination of Subjects Who Have Rejected Their Recovered Visualization as False Memories," *Issues in Child Abuse Accusations*, Vol. 6, 3 (1994), 125.
24. Composite of several cases.
25. Composite of several cases.
26. Pamela Freyd, "The False Memory Syndrome Foundation: Response to a Mental Health Crisis" (to appear in: Halperin, D.A. (Ed.), *False Memory Syndrome: Therapeutic and Forensic Perspectives*. American Psychiatric Press), 13.

Chapter 11. Angels of Light? The Spiritual Question

1. C. S. Lewis, *The Screwtape Letters*, (Uhrichsville, Ohio: Barbour and Company, 1982), 126.
2. Joe Salkowski, "A Different Diagnosis," the *Arizona Daily Star*, 5 December 1994, Section A, 9.
3. Ibid.
4. Jon Trott, "One Woman's Story," *Cornerstone*, Vol. 23, 106 (1995), 24.
5. C. S. Lewis, *The World's Last Night and Other Essays* (New York: Harcourt Brace Jovanovich, 1960), 5.
6. Jon Trott, "The Grade Five Syndrome," *Cornerstone*, 18.
7. Ibid.
8. Rossell Hope Robbins, *The Encyclopedia of Witchcraft and Demonology* (Crown Publishers, Inc., 1959), 310.
9. C. S. Lewis, *English Literature in the Sixteenth Century, Excluding Drama* (London: Oxford Universy Press, 1973).
10. C. S. Lewis, *Letters to Malcolm: Chiefly on Prayer* (New York: Harcourt Brace Jovanovich, 1964), 80.
11. C. S. Lewis, *God in the Dock: Essays on Theology and Ethics*, edited by Walter Hooper (Grand Rapids, Michigan: Eerdmans, 1970), 225.
12. C. S. Lewis, *The Problem of Pain* (New York: Macmillan, 1962), 127.

Chapter 12. Facing the Storm

1. Rossell Hope Robbins, *The Encyclopedia of Witchcraft and Demonology* (Crown Publishers, Inc., 1959), 2. Reprinted by permission of Crown Publishers, Inc.
2. Pamela Freyd, "The False Memory Syndrome Foundation: Response to a Mental Health Crisis" (to appear in: Halperin, D.A. (Ed.), *False Memory Syndrome: Therapeutic and Forensic Perspectives*. American Psychiatric Press), 15.
3. Headlines taken from various issues of the *FMS Foundation Newsletter*.
4. Ibid.
5. Ibid.
6. Ibid.
7. Ibid.
8. Ibid.
9. Ibid.
10. Ibid.
11. Ibid.
12. Ibid.
13. Ibid.
14. Ibid.
15. Ibid.
16. Rossell Hope Robbins, *The Encyclopedia of Witchcraft and Demonology*, 483.
17. Eric L. Nelson and Paul Simpson, "First Glimpse: An Initial Examination of Subjects Who Have Rejected Their Recovered Visualization as False Memories," *Issues in Child Abuse Accusations*, Vol. 6, 3 (1994), 125.
18. Personal communication from Dr. Chris Bardon to the author.
19. New Hampshire, State of. Hillsborough County Superior Court, *State of New Hampshire v. Joel Hungerford*, 94-045 thru 94-S-047, *State of New Hampshire v. John Morahan*, 93-S-1734 thru 93-S-1936 (1994), 1.
20. Personal communication from Dr. Paul McHugh to the author. Please see Paul R. McHugh, "Witches, Multiple Personalities, and Other Psychiatric Artifacts," *Nature Medicine*, 1(2) (February 1995), 110-114.
21. Rossell Robbins, *The Encyclopedia of Witchcraft and Demonology*, 17-18.
22. C. S. Lewis, *Christian Reflections*, edited by Walter Hooper (Grand Rapids, Mich.: Eerdmans, 1967), 111.

Appendix A. A Word to Regression Believers

1. C. S. Lewis, *God in the Dock: Essays on Theology and Ethics*, edited by Walter Hooper (Grand Rapids, Michigan: Eerdmans, 1970), 25-26.

About the Author

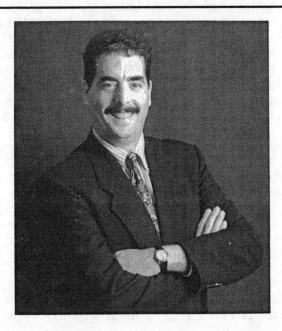

Dr. Paul Simpson is a psychologist, professional family mediator and former case manager with Child Protective Services who has worked extensively with victims of physical and sexual abuse, as well as sexual perpetrators. Dr. Simpson, a former practicing regressionist, began researching FMS and critiquing regression therapy in 1992 and founded *Project Middle Ground* in 1993 as a means of promoting dialogue between regression clients and their estranged families. This eventually expanded to include recovery and restoration work for "retractors." Through *Project Middle Ground*, Dr. Simpson has been instrumental in helping professionals and the general public have a better understanding of the FMS crisis. Offering hope, healing and clarity, he has been a driving force in assisting individuals and families to mediate their differences. In recognition of his professionalism he is listed in the *National Register of Health Care Providers in Psychology* and *Who's*

Who in Executives and Professionals. Dr. Simpson's expertise in the False Memory Crisis includes:

- Conducting FMS seminars nationally with professional groups since 1993.
- Establishing *Project Middle Ground*, the first program in the nation designed to mediate between regression clients and accused families.
- Helping retractors in healing from regression trauma, aiding them in understanding their FMS experiences, and reconciling with their families.
- Co-authored the first national study examining the experiences of retractors in the United States and Canada, which was published in 1994.
- Expert consultant to the Arizona Board of Psychologist Examiners.
- Member of a psychologists' special task force which is developing FMS and regression therapy policy for psychologists and therapists in the state of Arizona.
- Columnist and advisor for *Building Bridges*, the national newsletter for retractors.
- He has been interviewed on *Focus on the Family, Parent Talk Radio, Return to the Word, CNN, Frontline* (PBS), *The Leeza Gibbons Show,* and numerous magazines, newspapers and journals. In addition, he has provided consultation to *60 Minutes, Frontline, 20/20, Dateline,* and *The Oprah Winfrey Show.*

Dr. Simpson lives in Tucson, Arizona with his wife, Erin, and their two children, Maizie and Woody. If you would like to find out more about program services, set an appointment or arrange a seminar, you can do so by contacting Project Middle Ground staff at (520) 751-0101.